MASTERPIECES OF MEDICAL PHOTOGRAPHY

TWELVETREES PRESS

MASTERPIECES OF MEDICAL PHOTOGRAPHY

Selections from the Burns Archive

Edited by Joel-Peter Witkin

Captions by Stanley B. Burns, M.D.

TWELVETREES PRESS

1987

BELIEVING LIFE TO BE PASSION coupled with pain, I arranged to visit a major government archive in Washington D.C., an archive devoted to images of war. My hope was to find unknown photographic masterpieces from the American Civil War and publish the images in a book that would show the lunacy of hatred. After searching through thousands of photographs of mutilation and death, I was informed that my selections were not all original prints. The originals were part of a private collection of medical photographs belonging to Doctor Burns of New York City.

I met with Doctor Burns soon after and was greatly impressed with his passion for photographs relating to all facets of medicine. In a vaulted steel room, beneath the streets of Manhattan, Dr. Burns showed me not only the original prints I had sought, but many other unique daguerreotypes, ambrotypes, tintypes and paper prints from his vast collection of medical photography. These images, and others I studied in subsequent meetings, were a human, historic and cultural treasure; masterpieces.

Why did I consider them so? Not because they had survived time. A stone does as much. But because from the archaic past had survived an impulse, a transference of consciousness from one living being to another, emotional need becoming physical form. A masterpiece is part of that history of Creation. It has nothing to do with the history of taste and everything to do with achieving the highest knowledge of ourselves.

The work of painters and sculptors, regardless of content, must finally be presented as works of the imagination. It is only in our epoch that we possess the permanent mirror of memory we call photography, the most truthful presentation of reality ever known. Yet we continue to fear its darker images of ourselves, even from the past. The photographs presented here are not pre-Raphaelite fictional tableaux, nor surreal evocations of the paradisiacal. They are gifts to life, from another time to our own. The camera has given us the means to see ourselves in others, ourselves harmed, unloved, deformed, even dead. These images are triumphant contributions in the evolution of the quest for our highest attainment, to unselfishly help and heal one another, to eradicate all disease, both social and pathological.

Joel-Peter Witkin, 1987

1

Physician With His Medical Bag
L. Chilton, New York City
2½ x 3¼", Daguerreotype
c. 1847

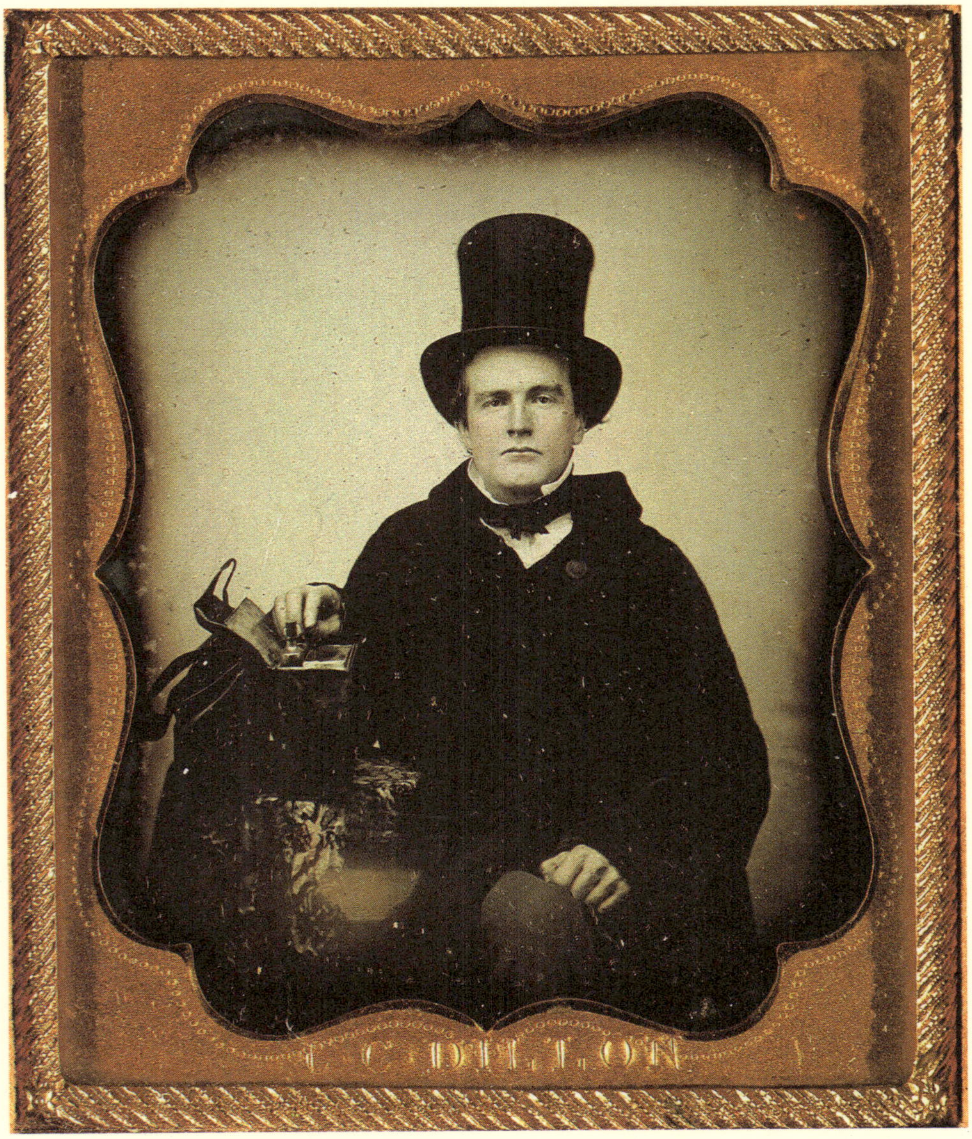
T. C. DILLON

2

Dissection Scene
Byron Reed, Kokimo, Indiana
8½ x 6½", Tintype of Daguerreotype
c. 1844

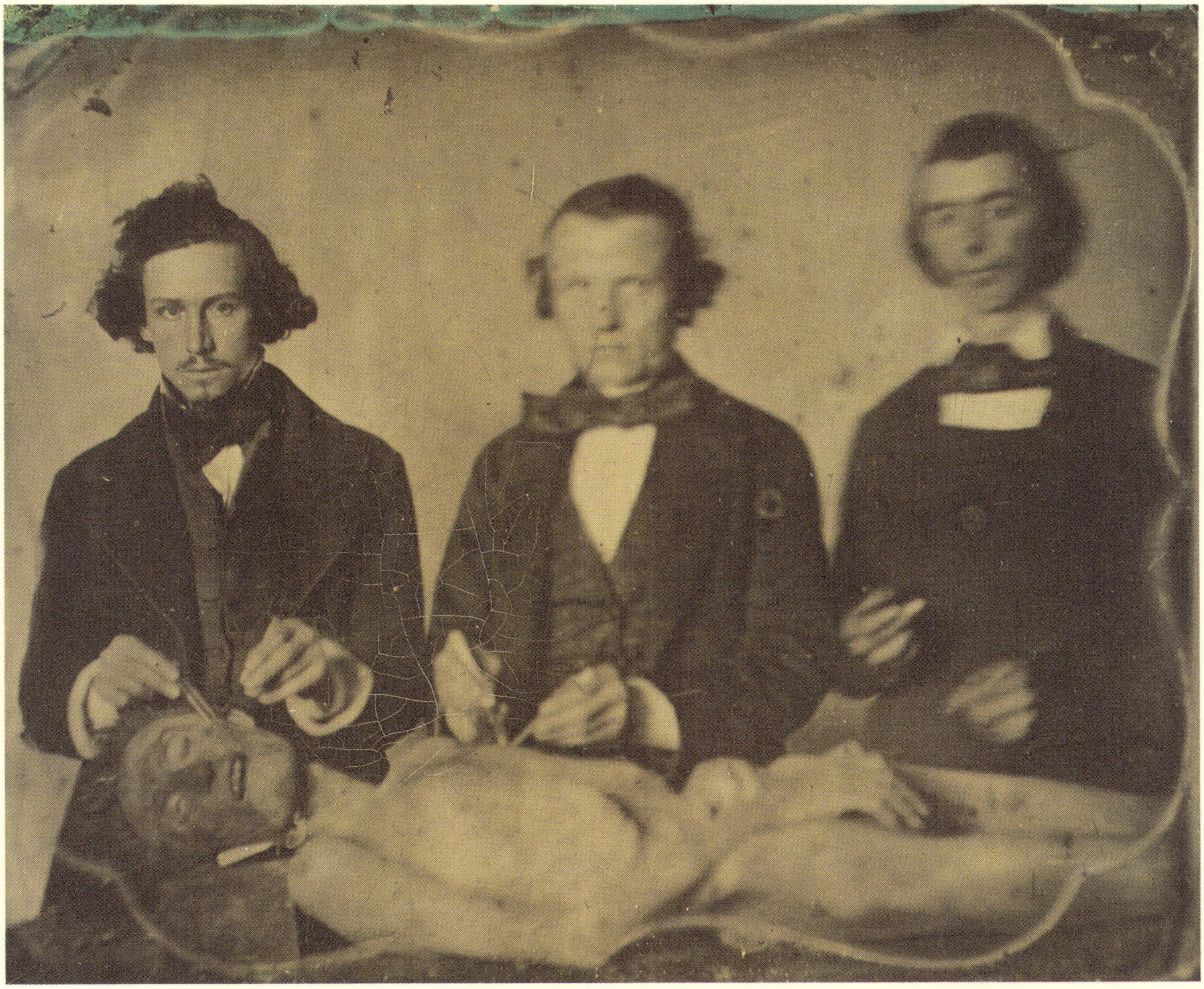

3

DR. LETTERMAN EXAMINING A PATIENT
Anonymous, Philadelphia
4¼ x 3¼", Daguerreotype
1849

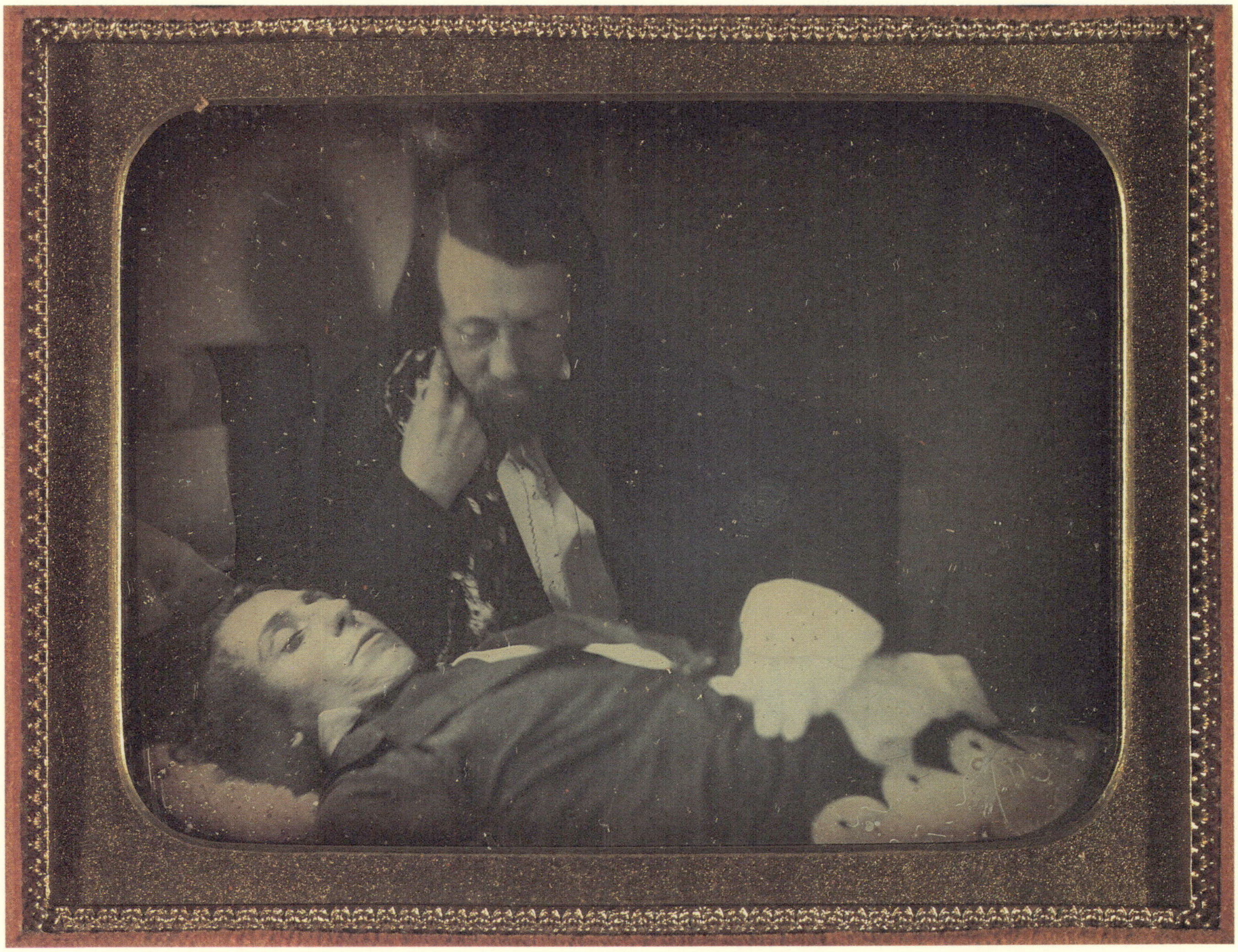

4

South American Indian With a Tumor of the Jaw
Anonymous, Caracas, Venezuela
3¼ x 4¼", Daguerreotype
1848

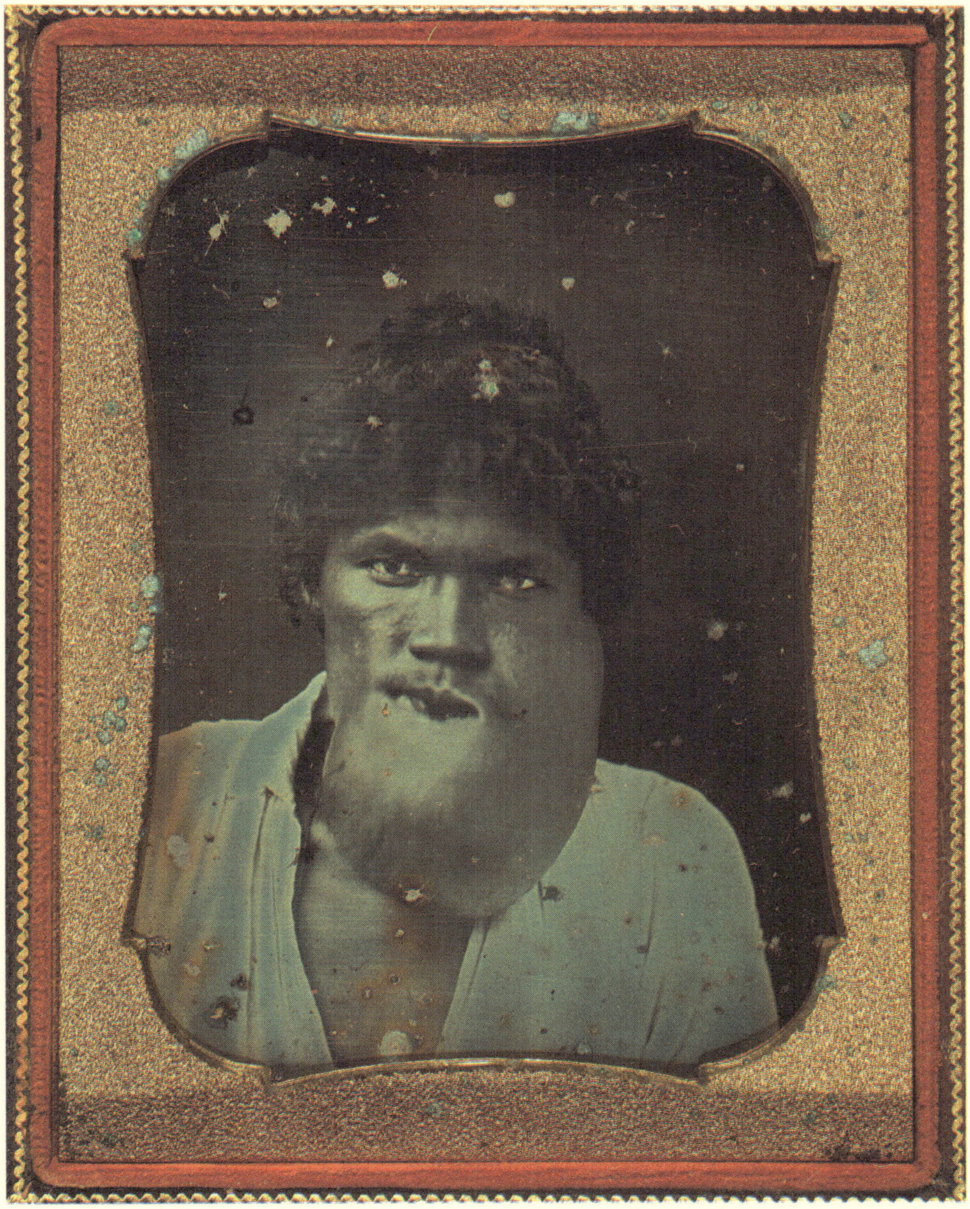

5

Mother With Her Dead Twins
Anonymous, United States
2¾ x 3¼″, Ambrotype
c. 1855

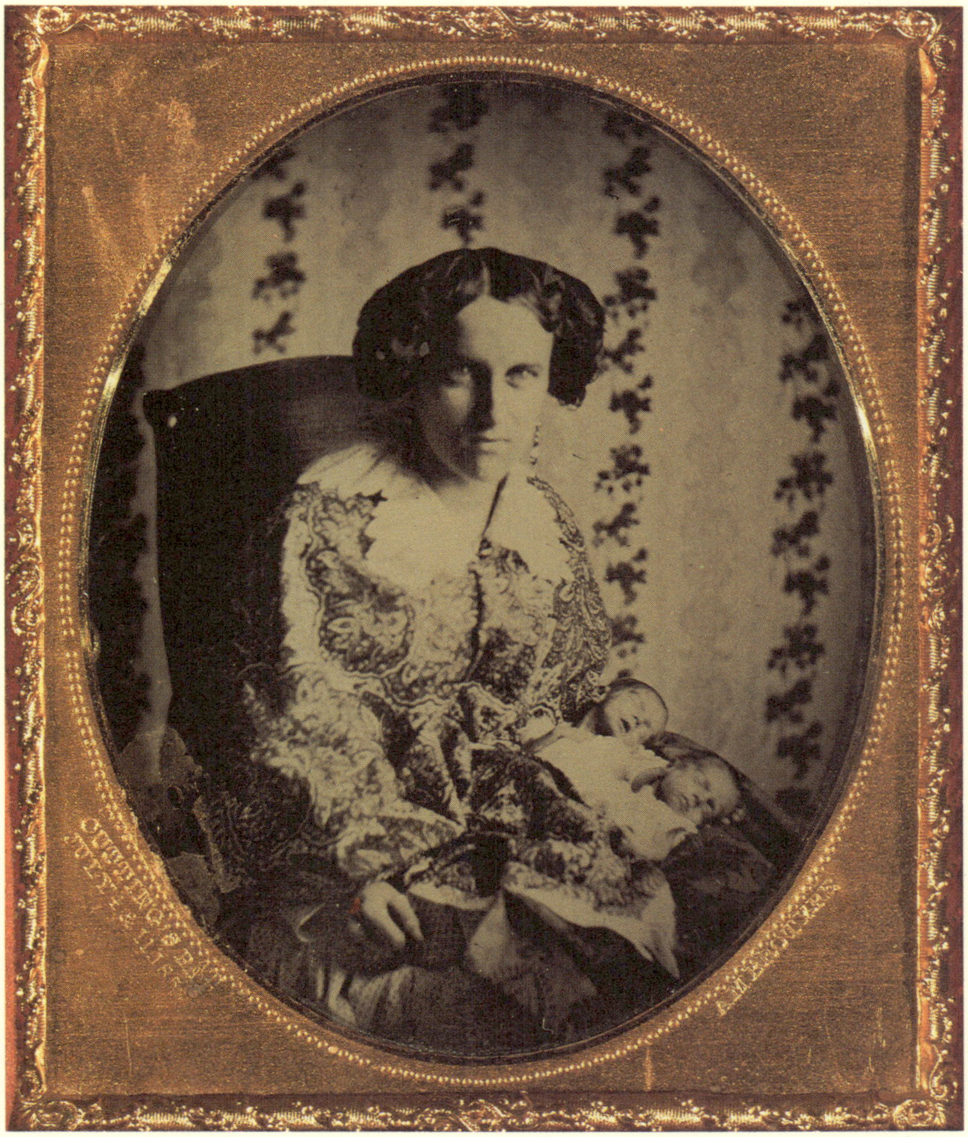

6

Dr. Sayre and His Suspension Device for Scoliosis
Anonymous, London
3½ x 4½", Albumen Print
1877

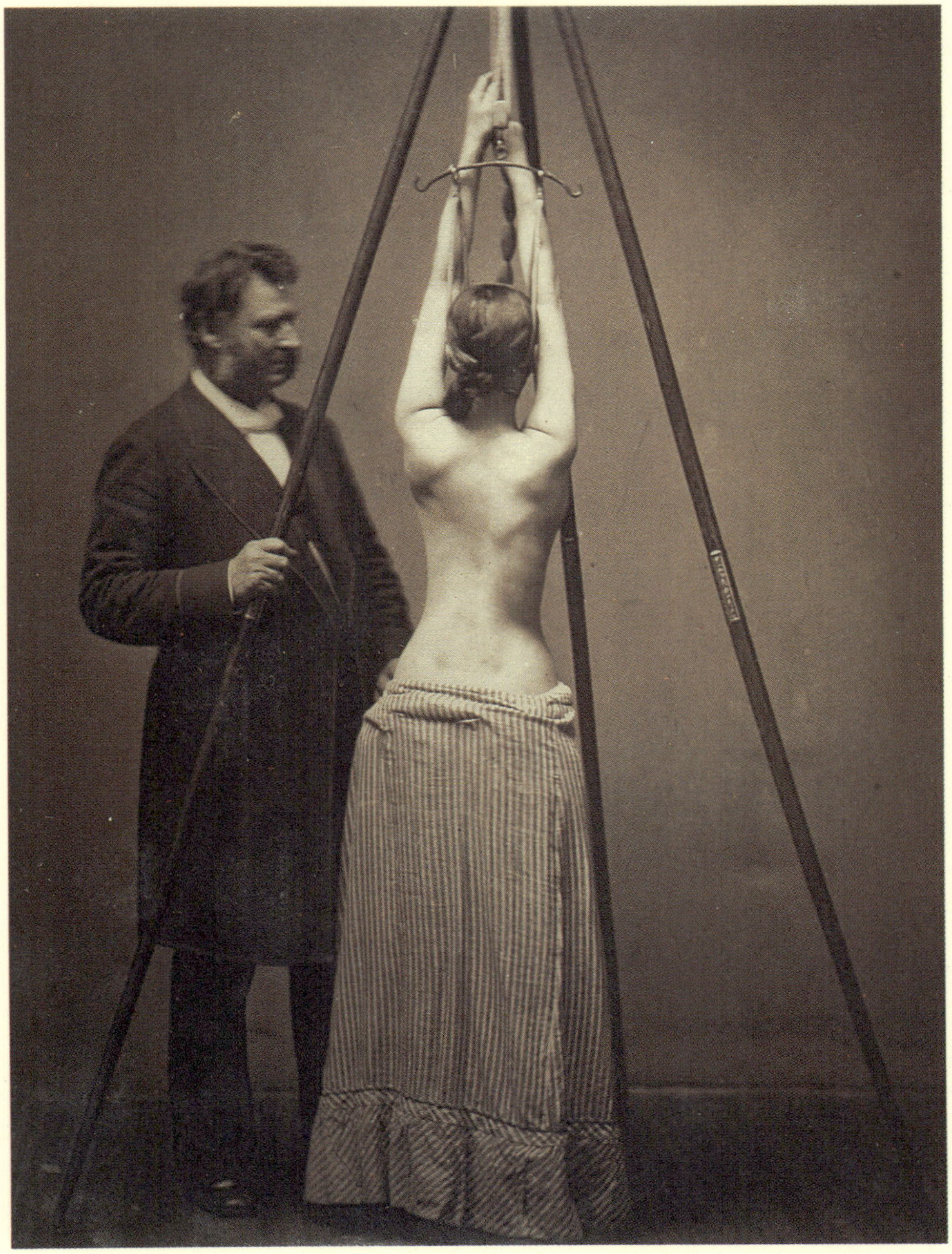

7

BERNHEIM'S HYPNOTIC TECHNIQUE
Anonymous, Chicago
3¼ x 3¼", Gelatin Print
c. 1895

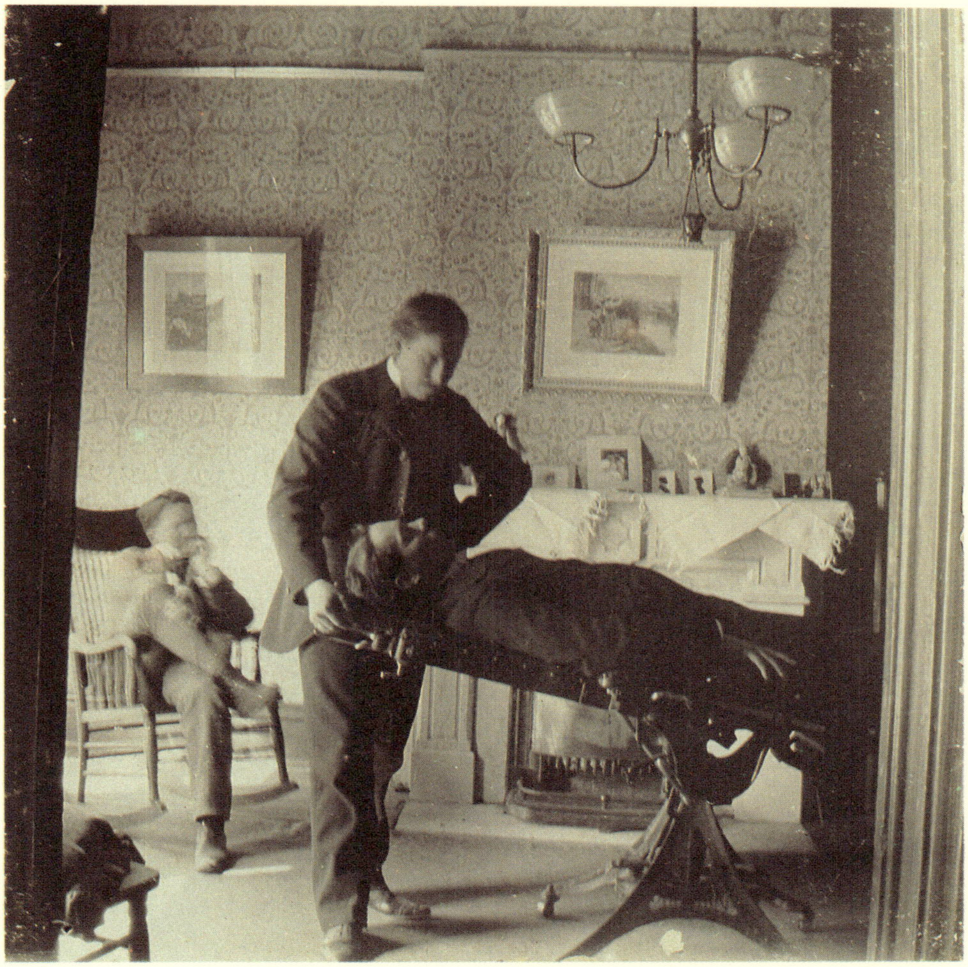

8

BLIND JAPANESE SHIATZU MASSAGE HEALER
Anonymous, Japan
2¼ x 4″, Carte de Visite, Tinted Albumen Print
c. 1860

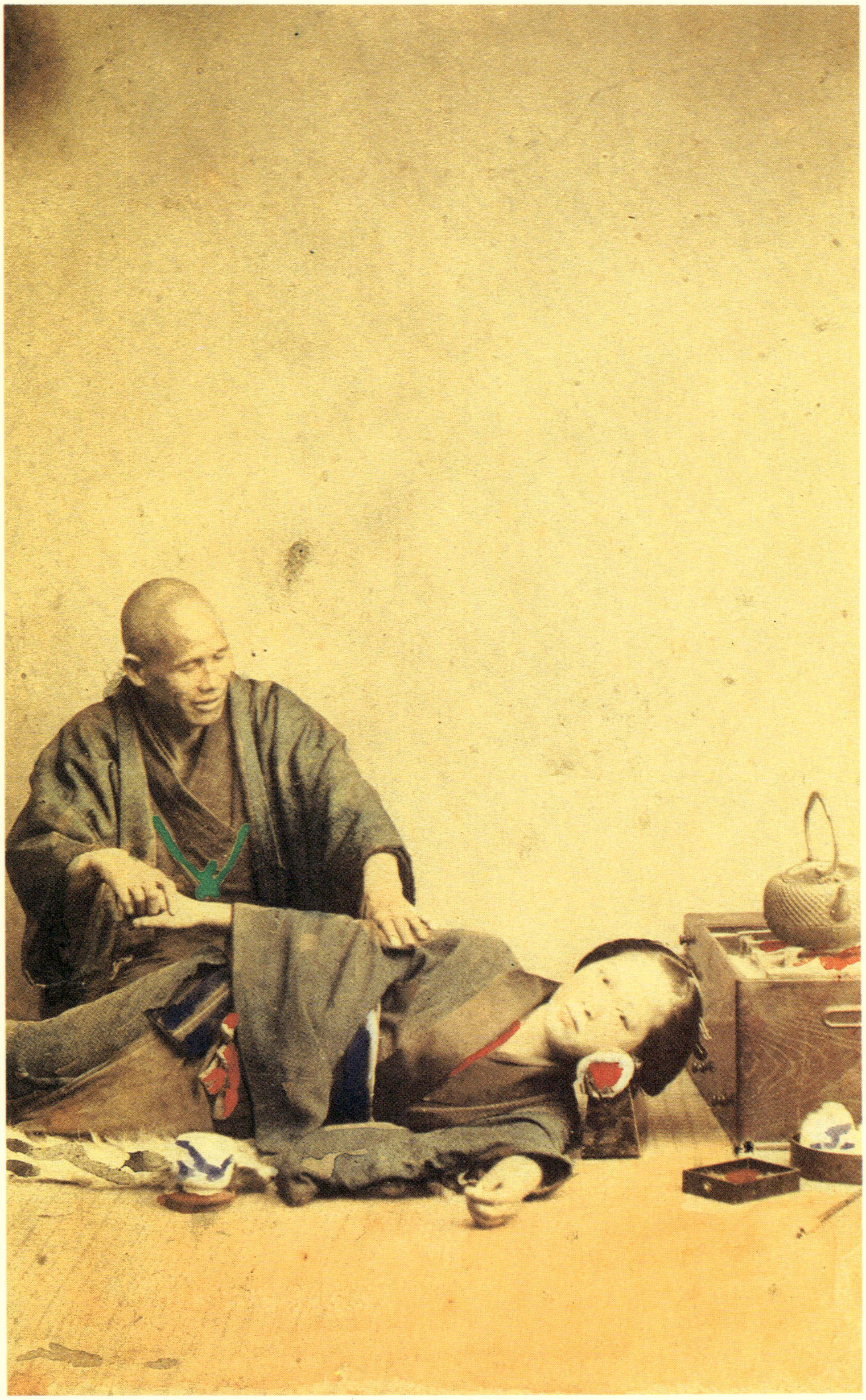

9

Psychiatric Patient in Rag Clothing
Anonymous, France
3½ x 5″, Silver Print
c. 1890

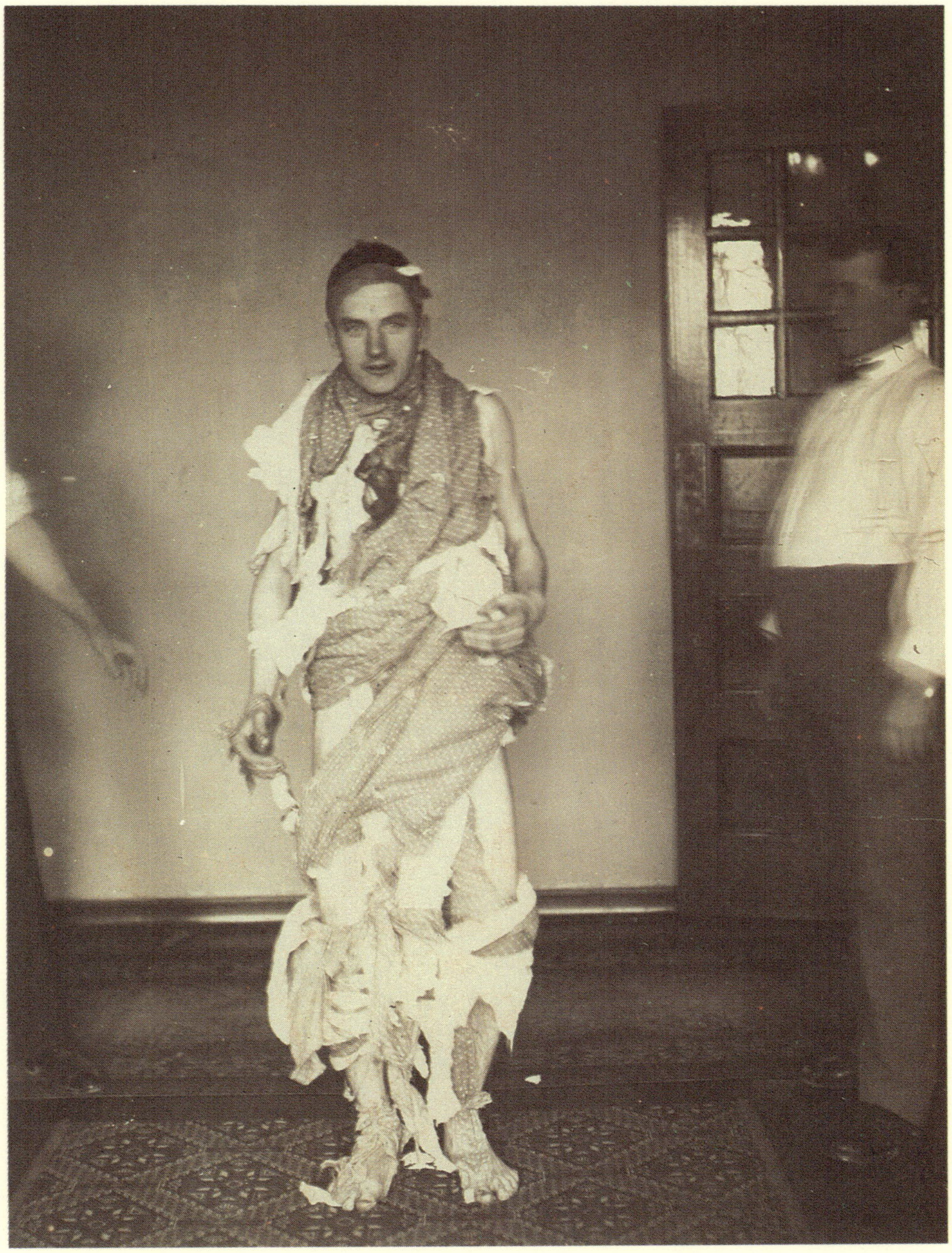

10

Muybridge Study of Human Motion
Eadweard Muybridge, United States
8½ x 14¼", Heliotype
1887

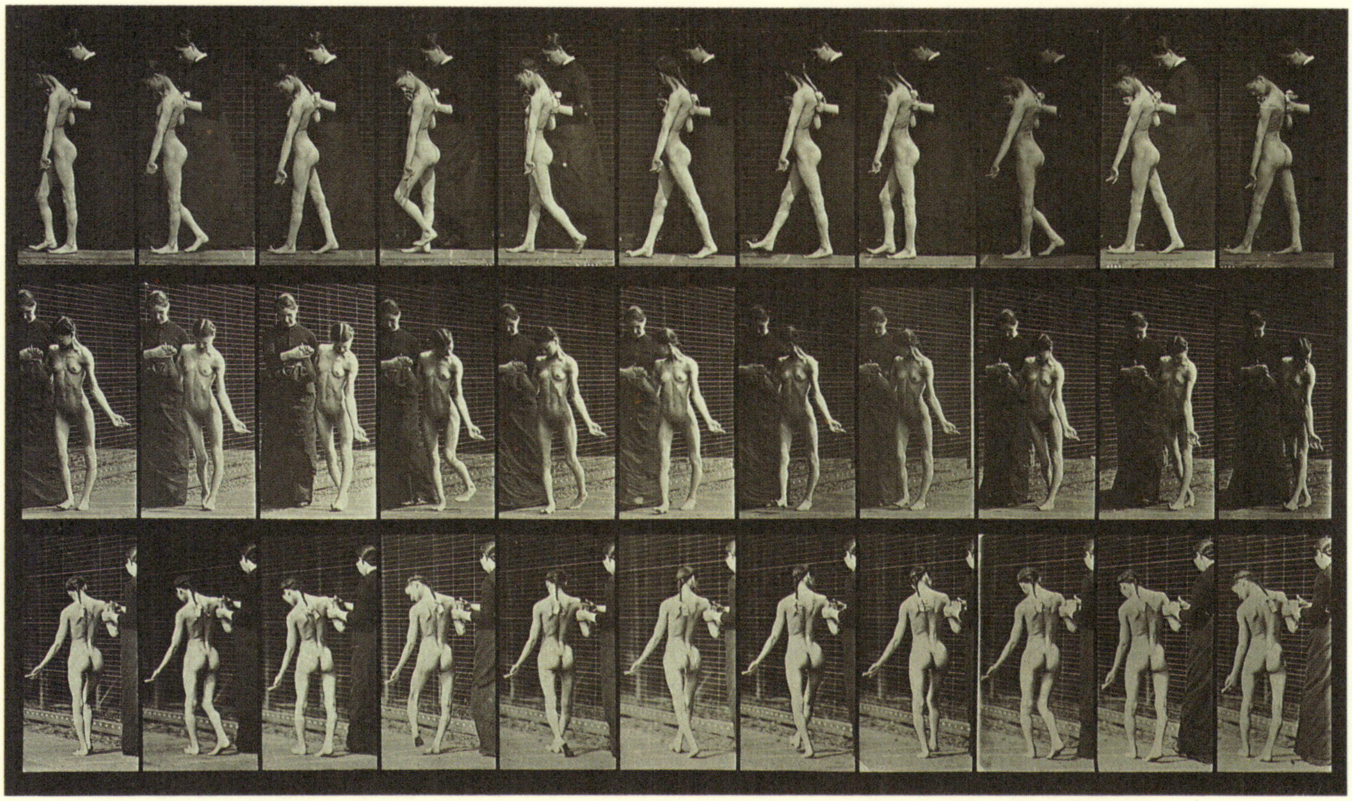

11

DR. AZOUX AND HIS MEDICAL MANNEQUIN
Bisson Freres, France
2¼ x 4″, Carte de Visite, Albumen Print
c. 1859

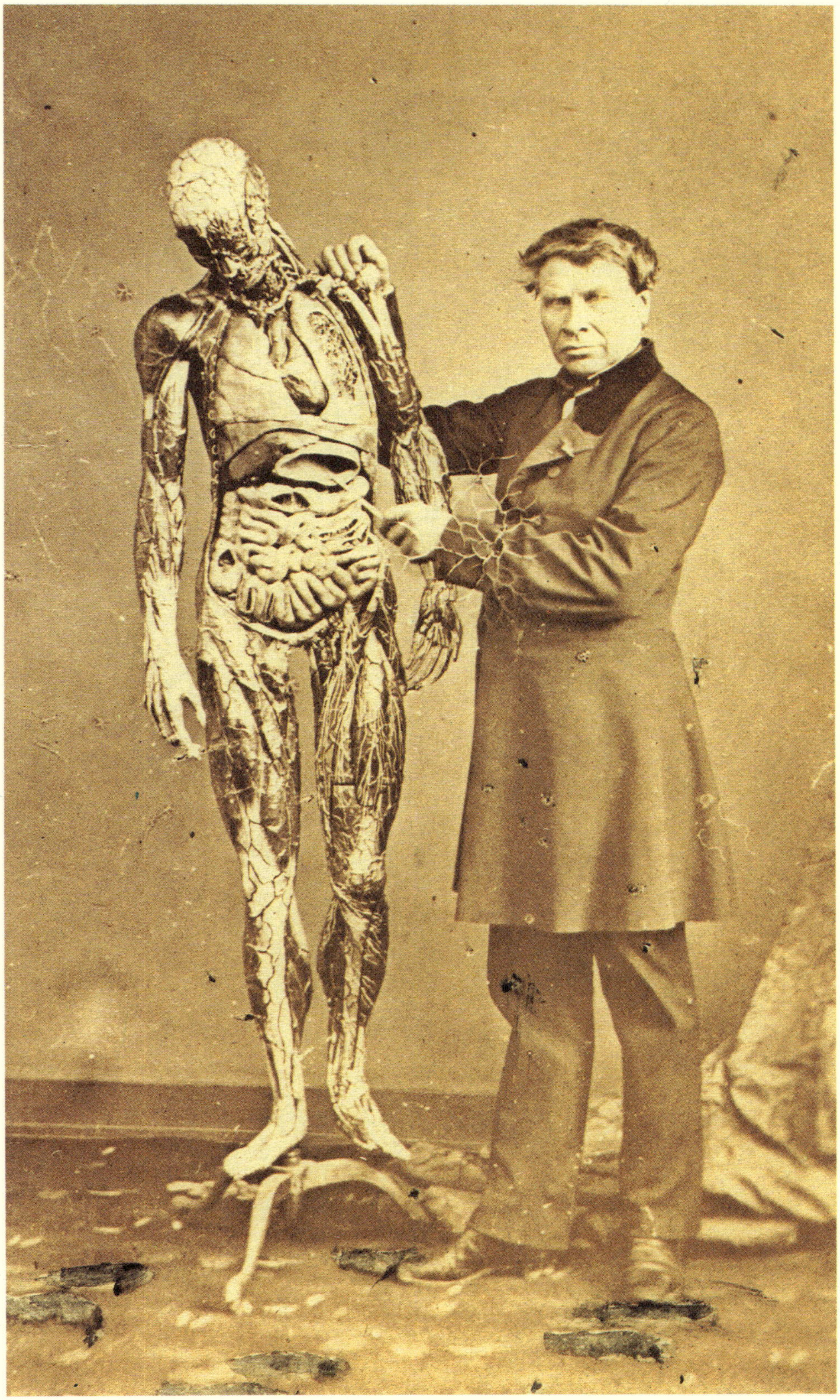

12

Old Woman With Eye Tumor
Anonymous, United States
4¼ x 5½″, Albumen Print
c. 1878

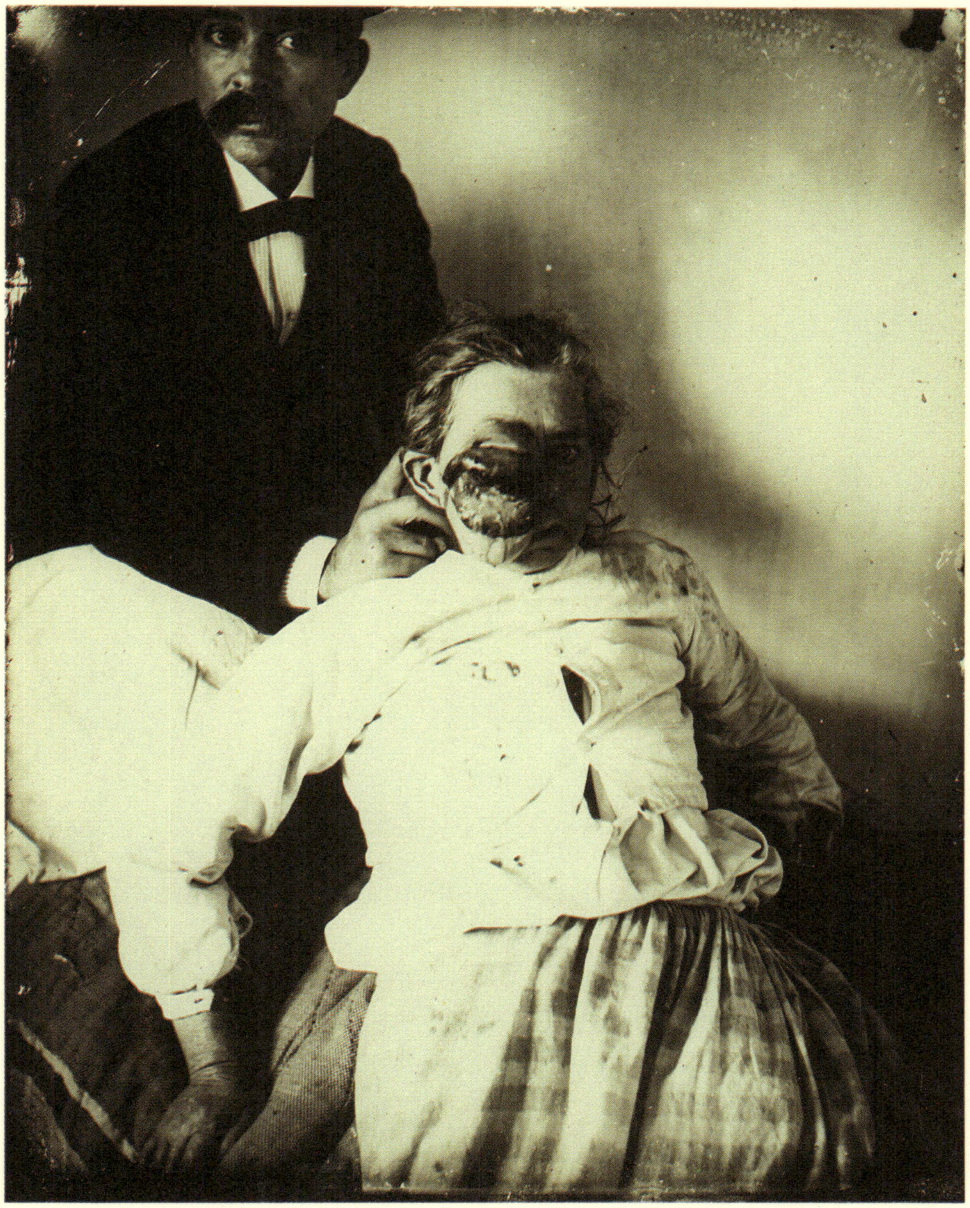

13

Dissected Head In Soup Plate
Howard Brundage, M.D., Columbus, Ohio
7 x 5″, Silver Print
1905

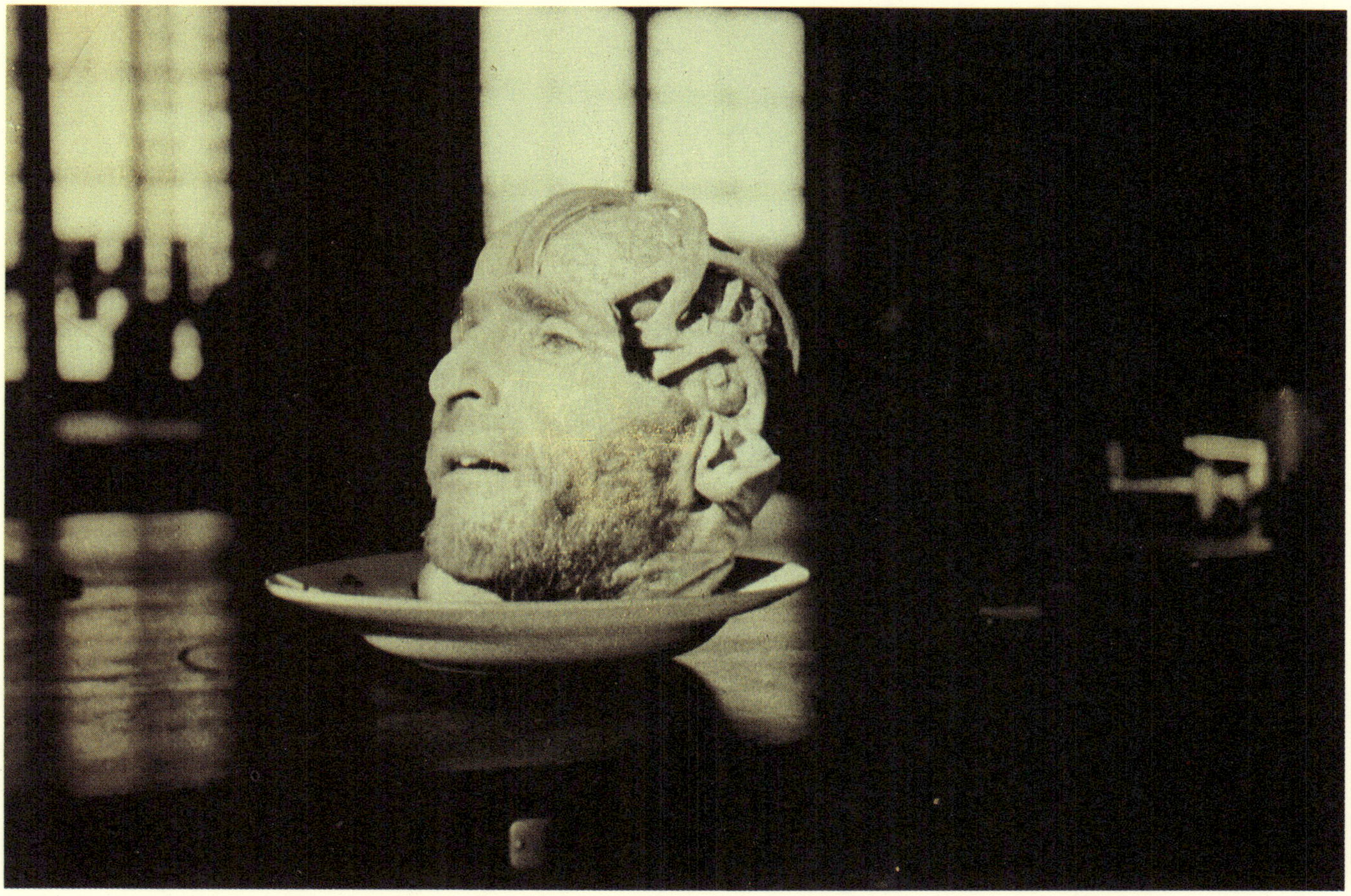

14

Young Woman With Elephantiasis From Scarlet Fever
O.G. Mason, New York City
4 x 6¼″, Artotype
1878

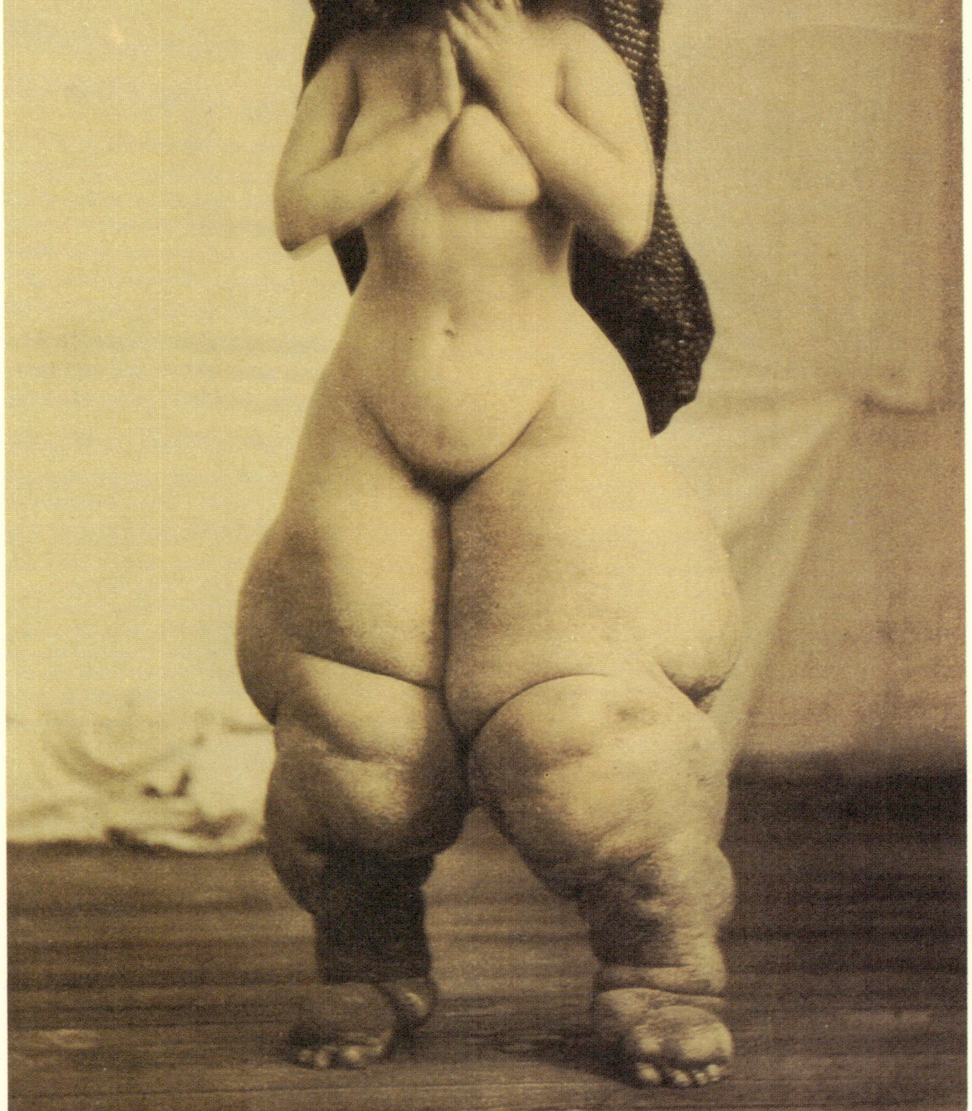

15

Erysipelas Infection After Thumb Amputation
Reed B. Bontecou, M.D., Washington D.C.
3½ x 3½", Albumen Print
1865

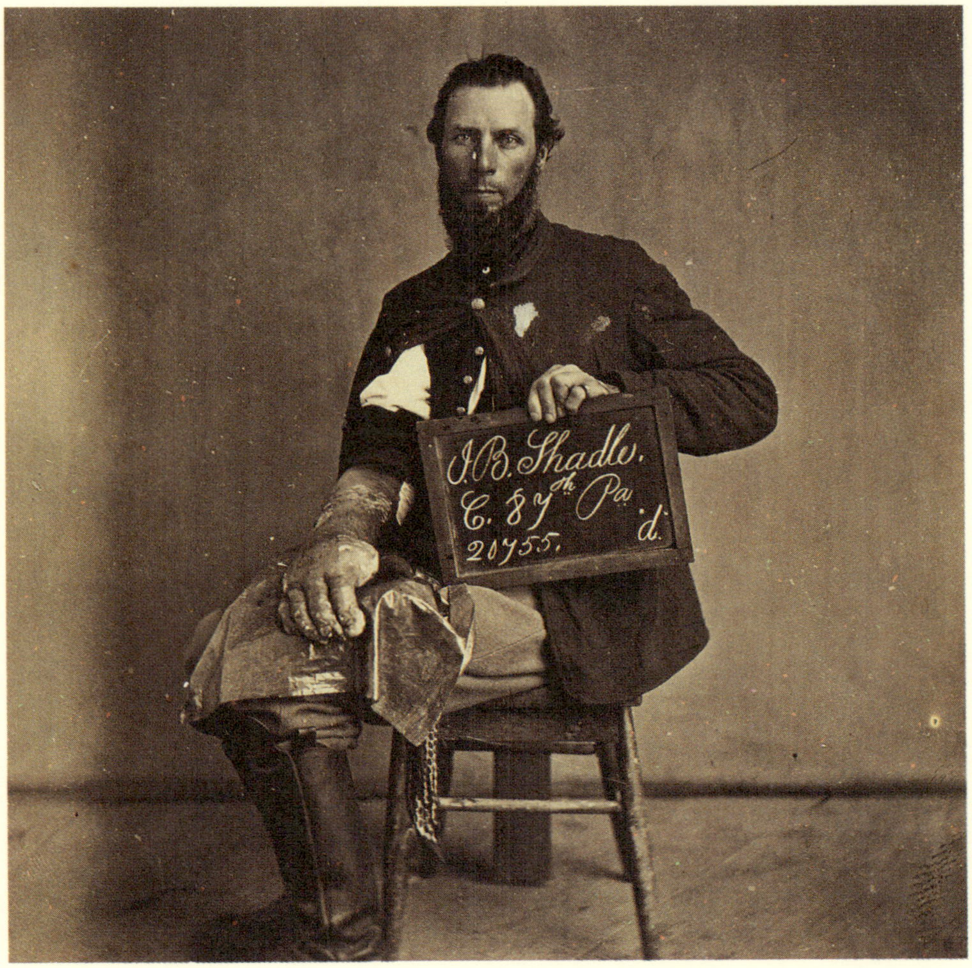
J.B. Shadle.
C. 87th Pa.
20755.
d.

16

Hospital Gangrene
Reed B. Bontecou, Washington D.C.
4½ x 6½", Albumen Print
1865

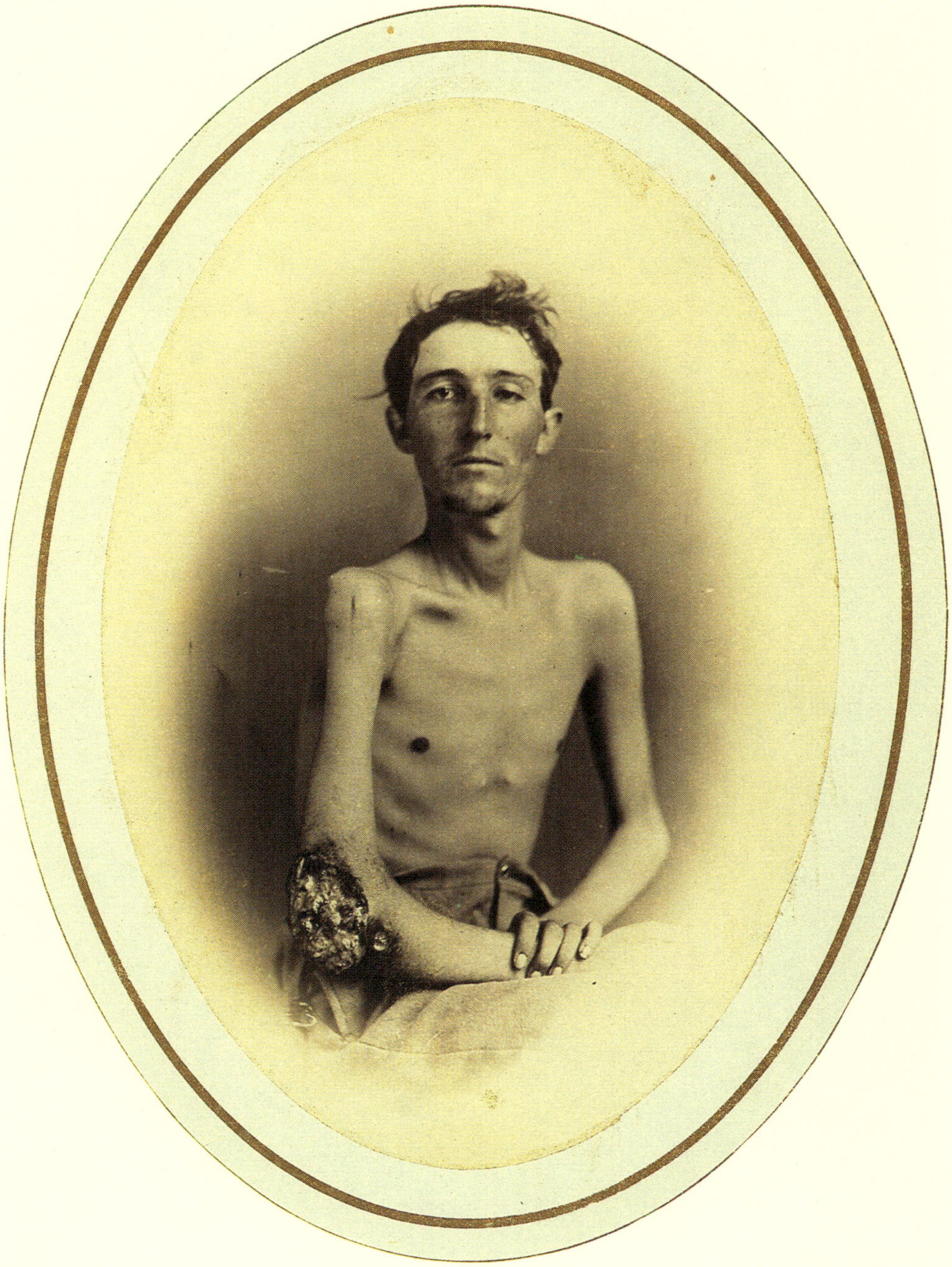

17

Sutured Gunshot Wound of the Upper Arm
Reed B. Bontecou, M.D., Washington D.C.
4½ x 6½", Albumen Print
1865

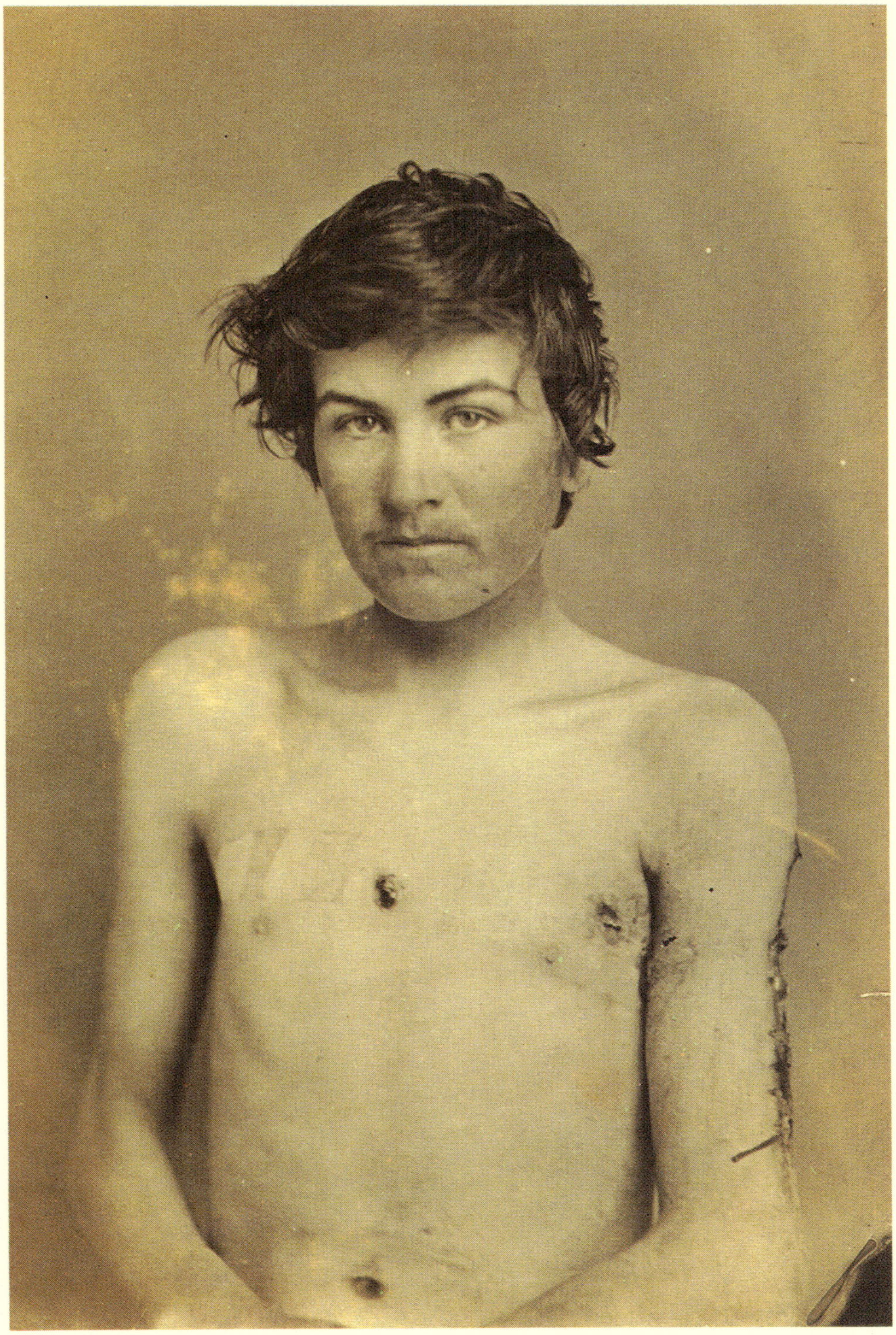

18

Amputation at the Hip Joint
Reed B. Bontecou, M.D., Washington D.C.
4½ x 6½", Albumen Print
1865

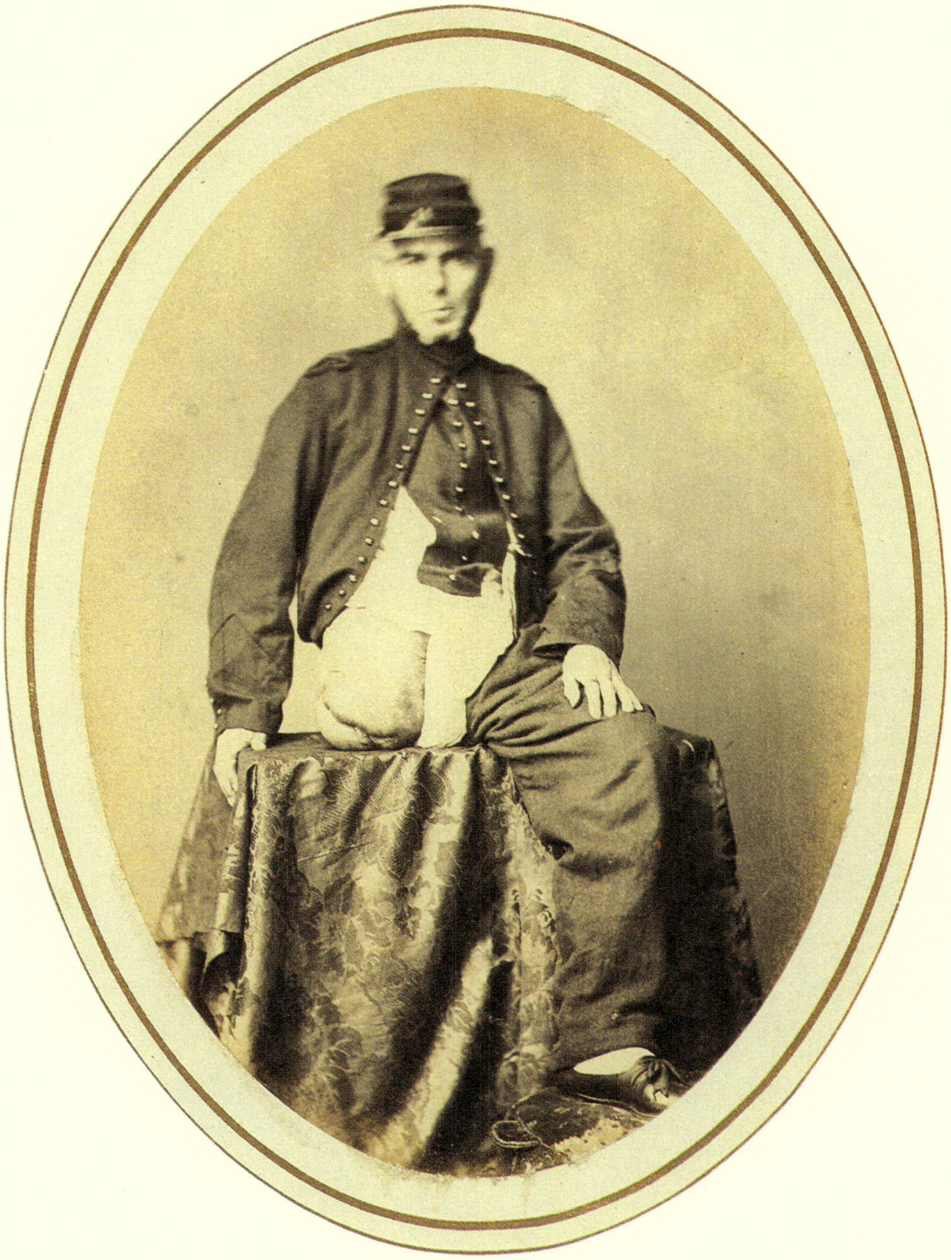

19

Gunshot Wound of the Hand
Reed B. Bontecou, M.D., Washington D.C.
4½ x 6½", Albumen Print
1865

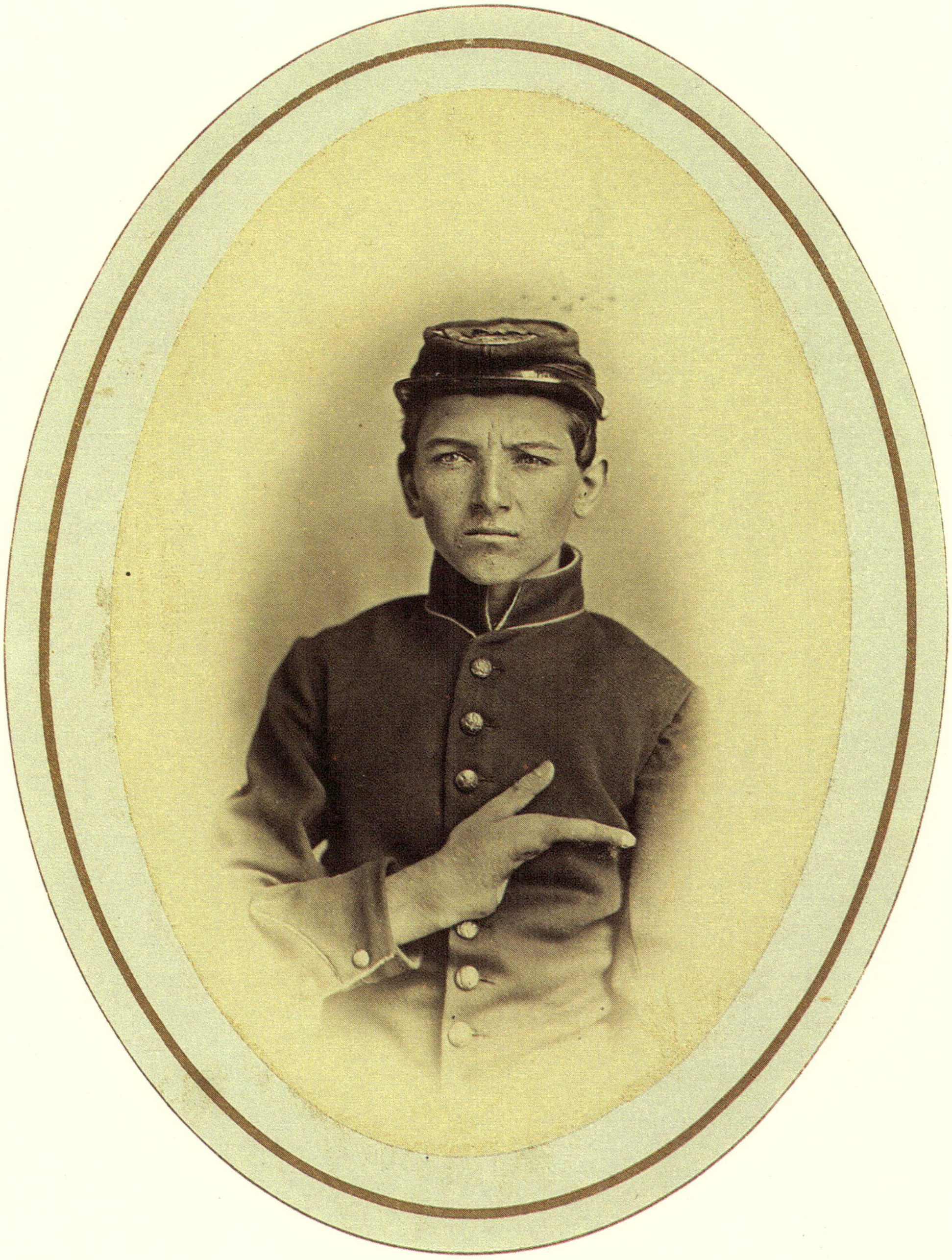

20

ARM AMPUTATION BY FLAP TECHNIQUE
Reed B. Bontecou, M.D., Washington D.C.
4½ x 6½", Albumen Print
1865

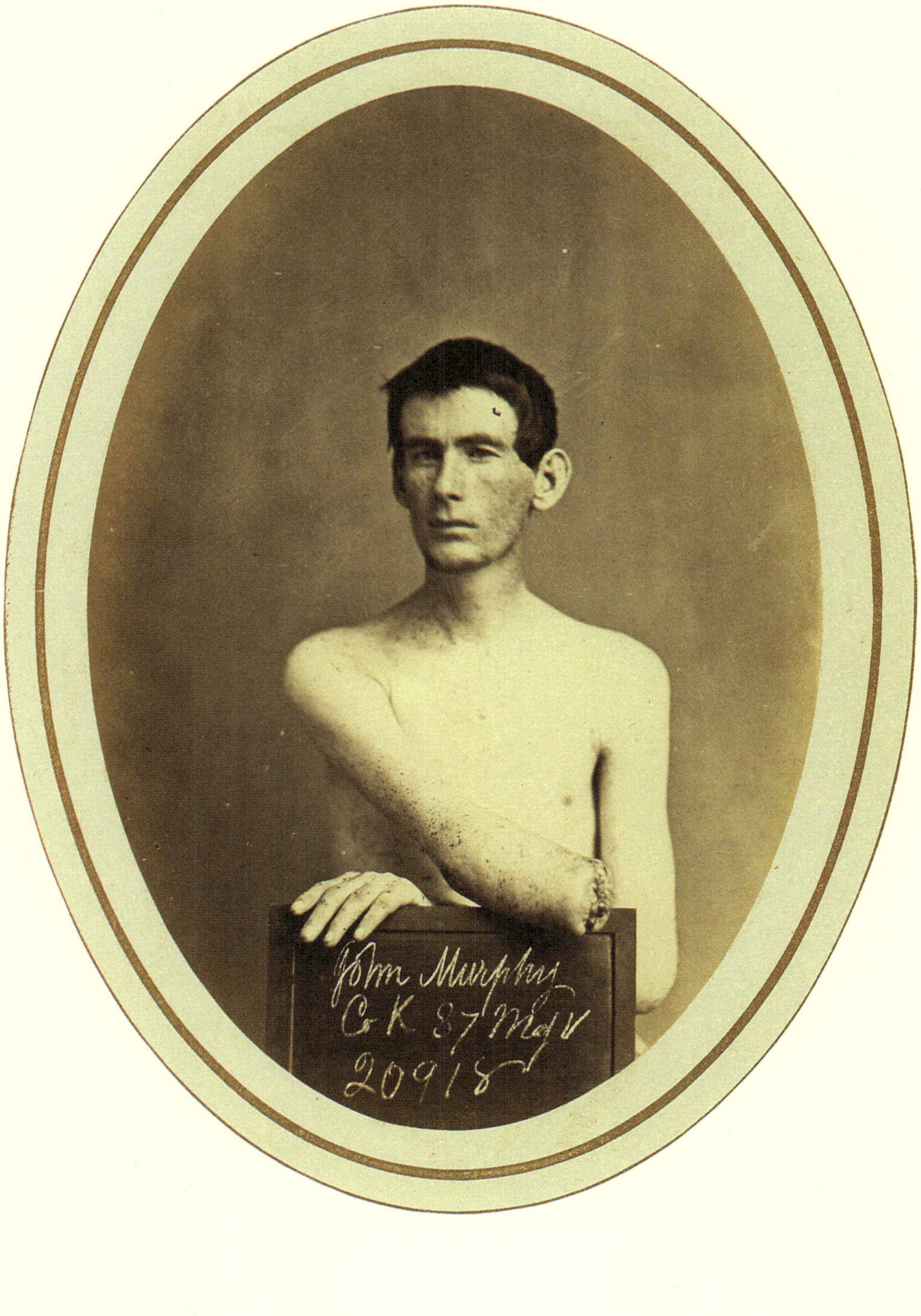

John Murphy
Co K 87 NyV
20918

21

Bone Excision
Reed B. Bontecou, M.D., Washington D.C.
4½ x 6½″, Albumen Print
1864

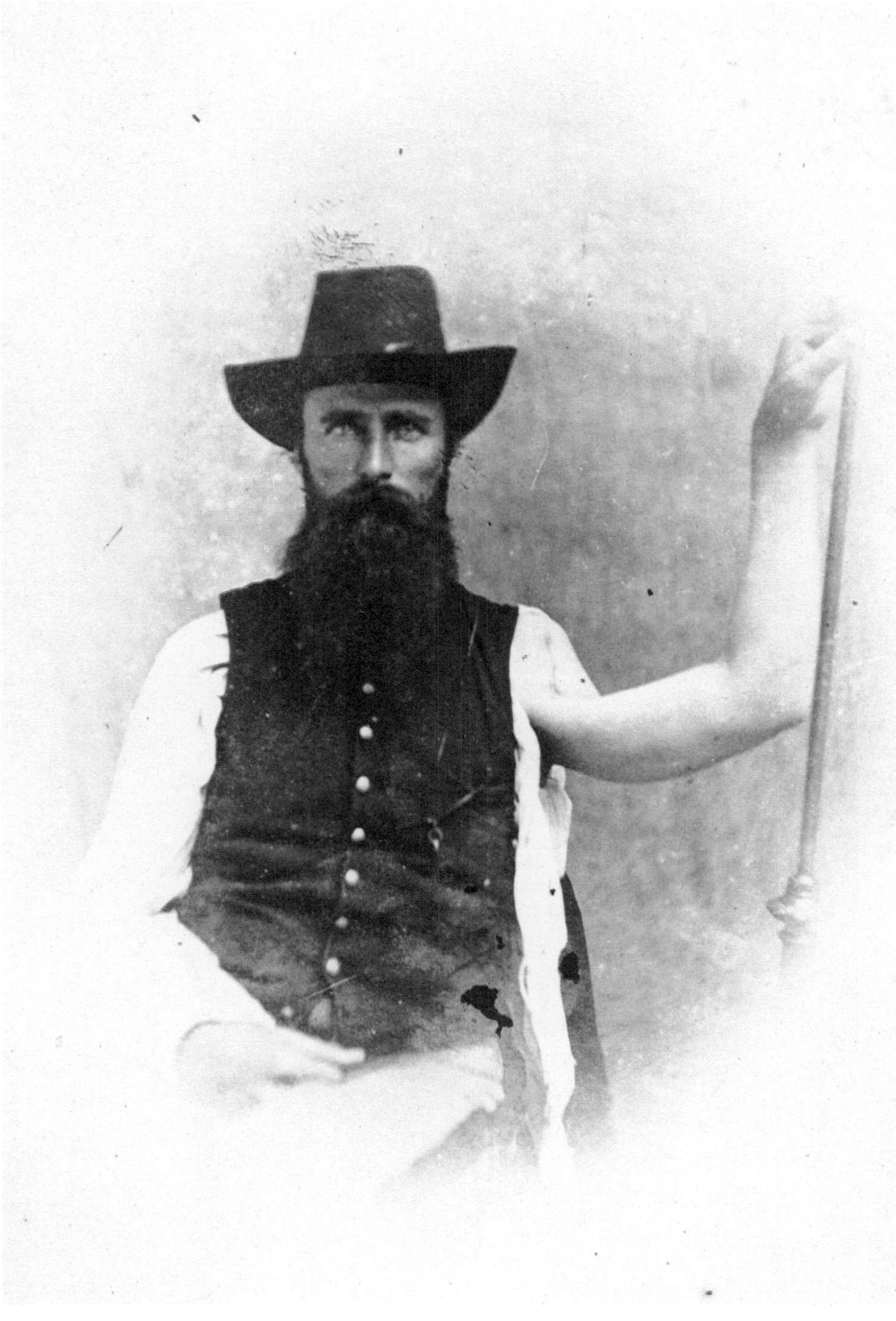

22

GUNSHOT WOUND OF THE HEAD
Reed B. Bontecou, M.D., Washington D.C.
4½ x 6½", Albumen Print
1865

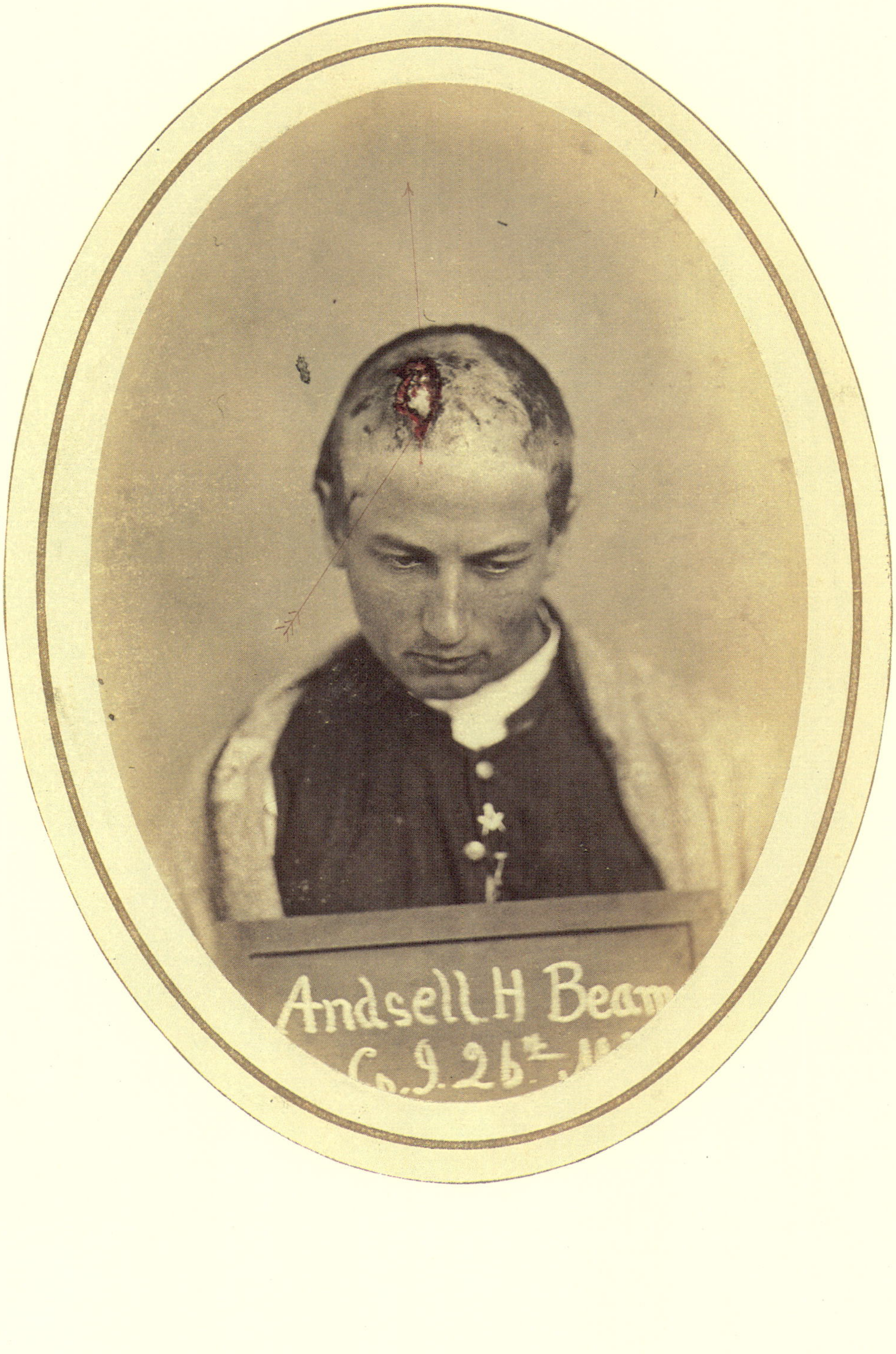
Andsell H Beam
Co. I. 26th

23

EMBALMING SURGEON
Matthew Brady
3¼ x 3¼″, Albumen Print
1864

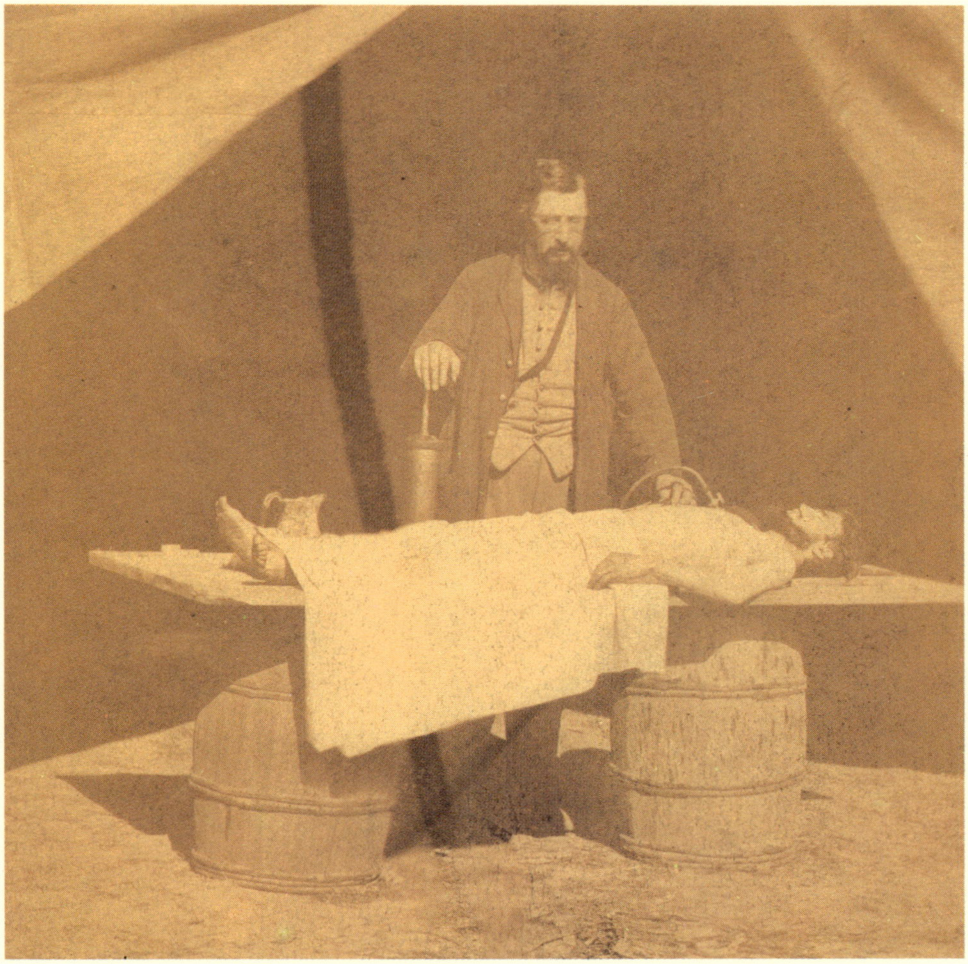

24

A Morning's Work
Reed B. Bontecou, M.D., Washington D.C.
6 x 4″, Albumen Print
1865

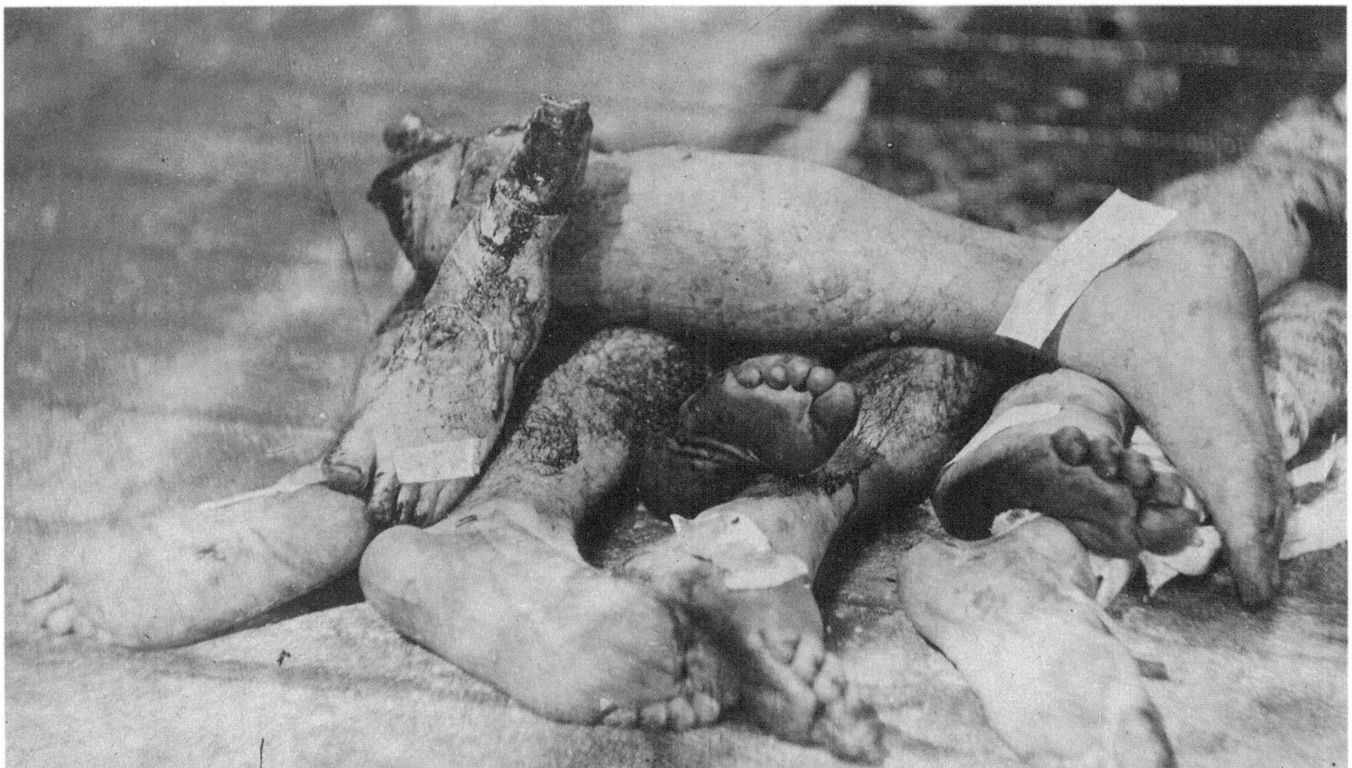

25

Andersonville Prisoner
Matthew Brady, Washington D.C.
3 1/4 x 3 1/4", Albumen Print
c. 1865

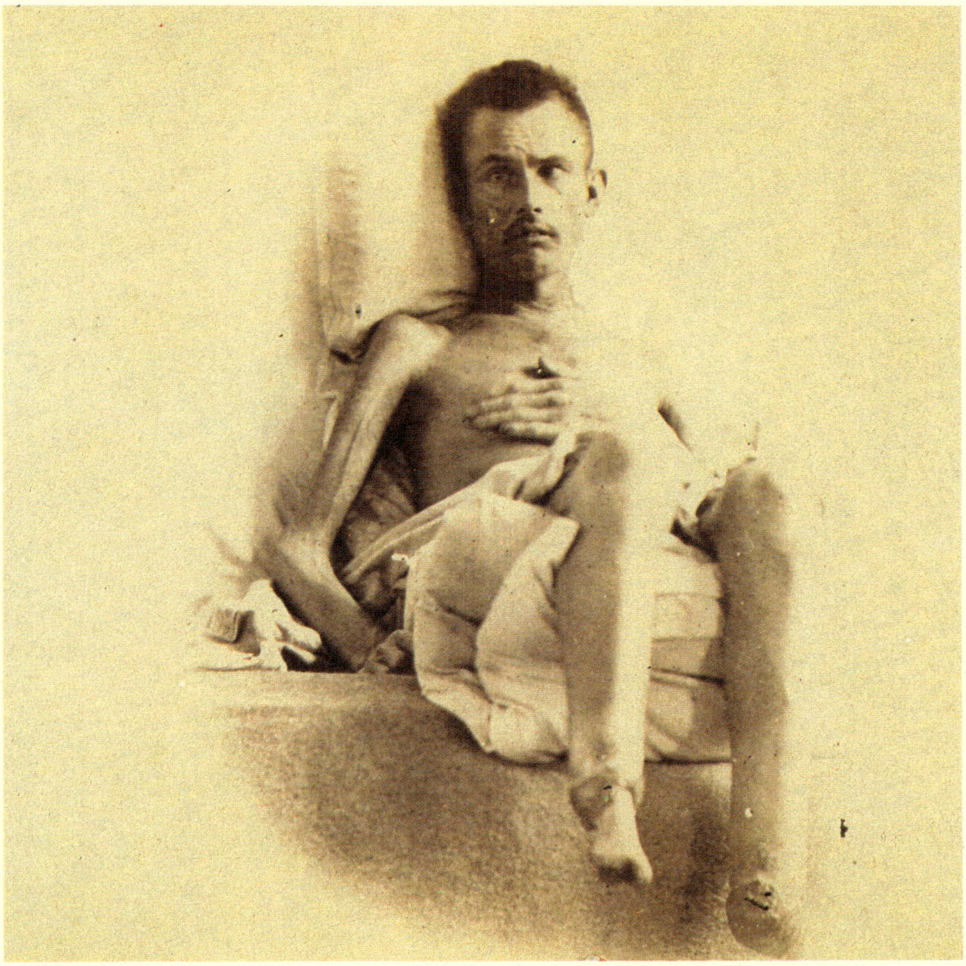

26

BONE FRAGMENTS
Reed B. Bontecou, M.D., Washington D.C.
2¼ x 4″, Carte de Visite, Albumen Prints
1864

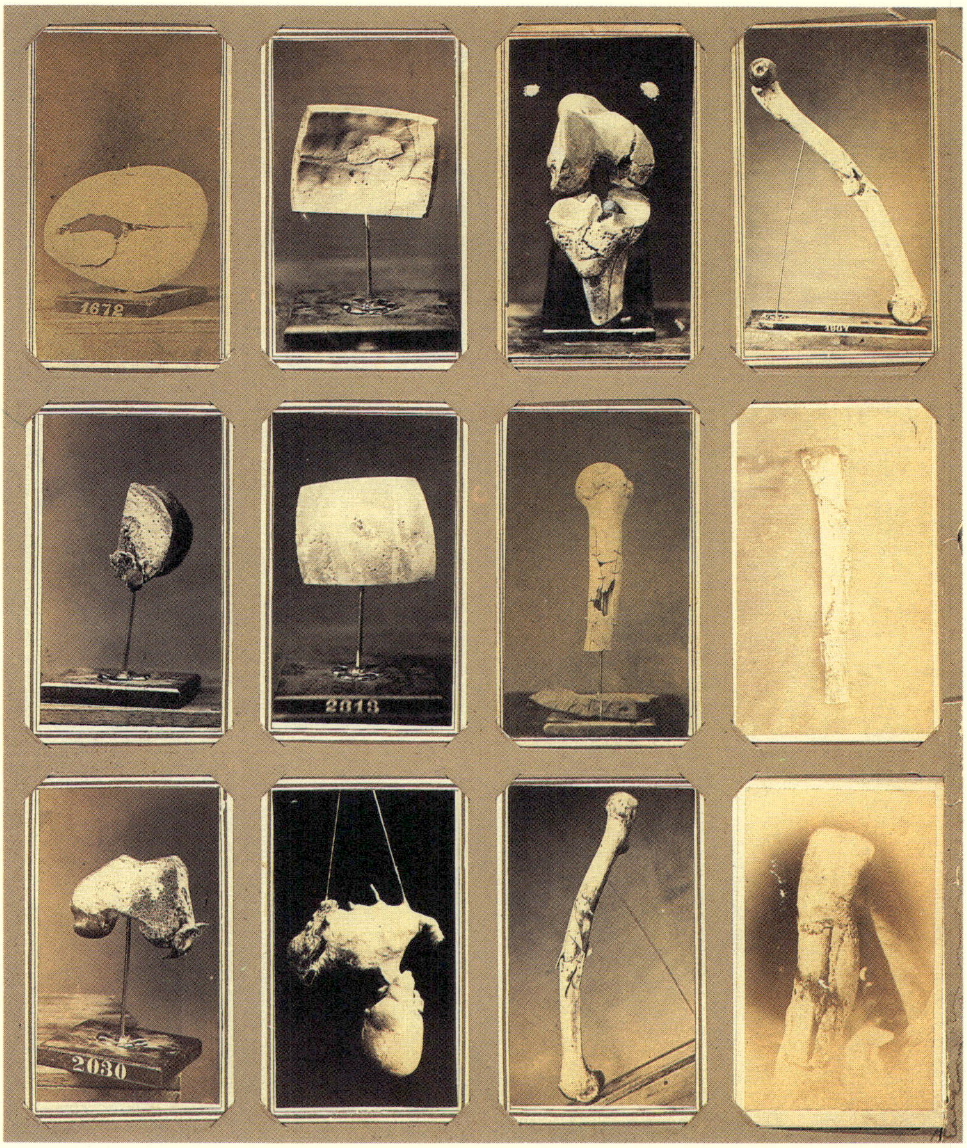
1672
2030

27

WOMAN WITH NECK LESIONS
O.G. Mason, New York City
4¾ x 6¼", Artotype
c. 1881

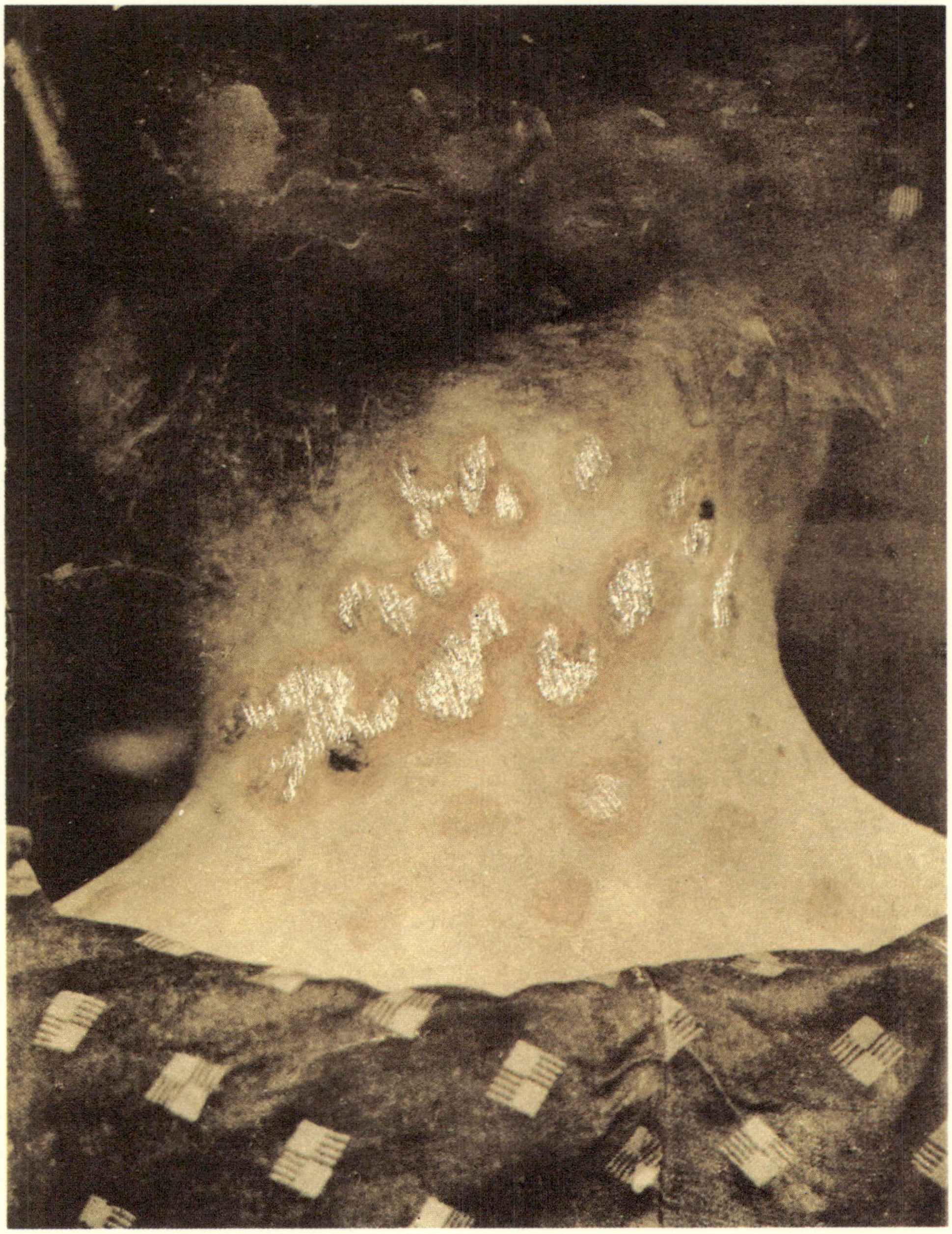

28

Girl With Large Foot Jumping Rope
Dewitt, Scranton, Pennsylvania
4 x 5½″, Cabinet Card
c. 1895

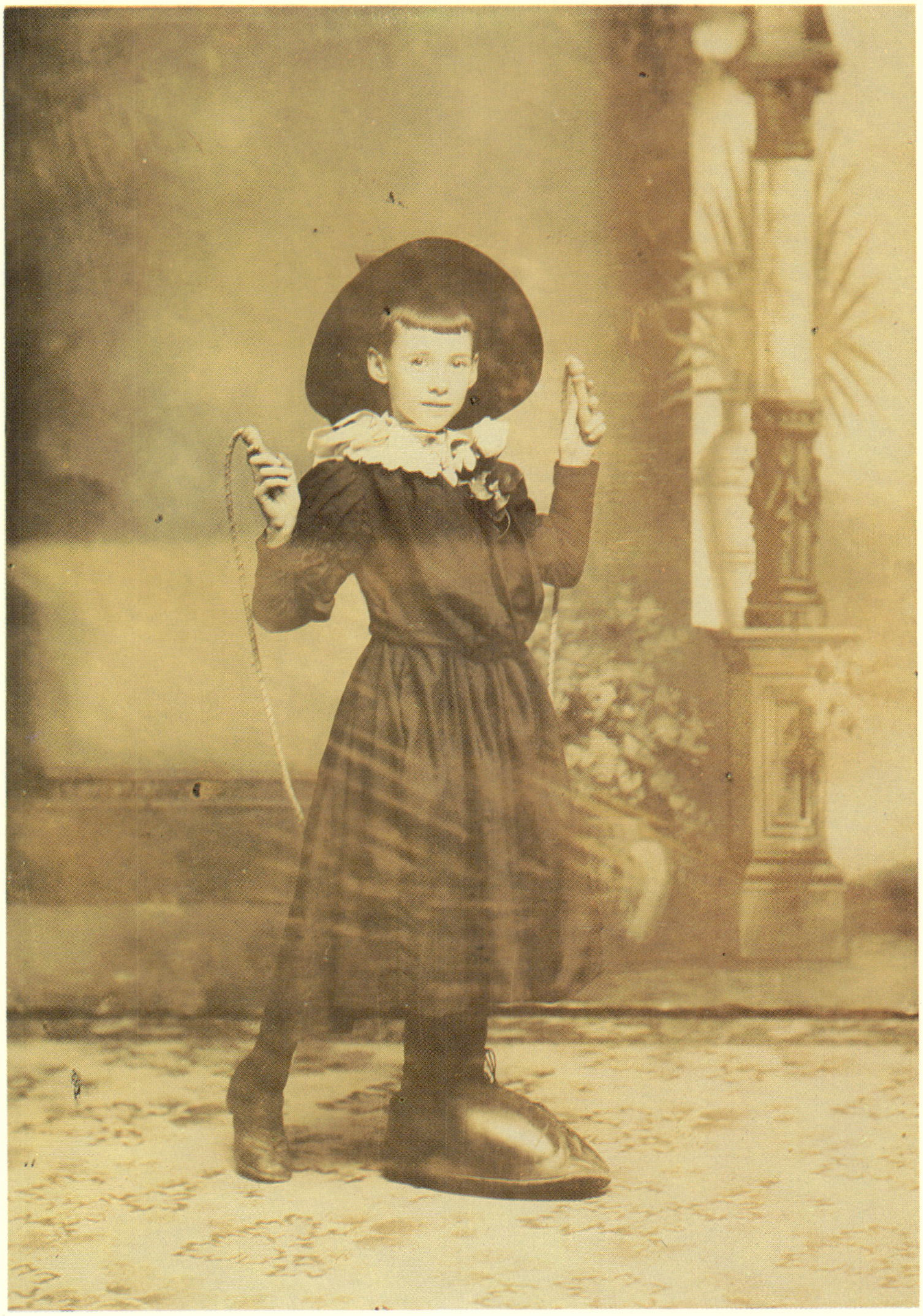

29

Amputated Arm Cured By Earth Dressing
Anonymous, Philadelphia
3 x 4″, Albumen Print
1869

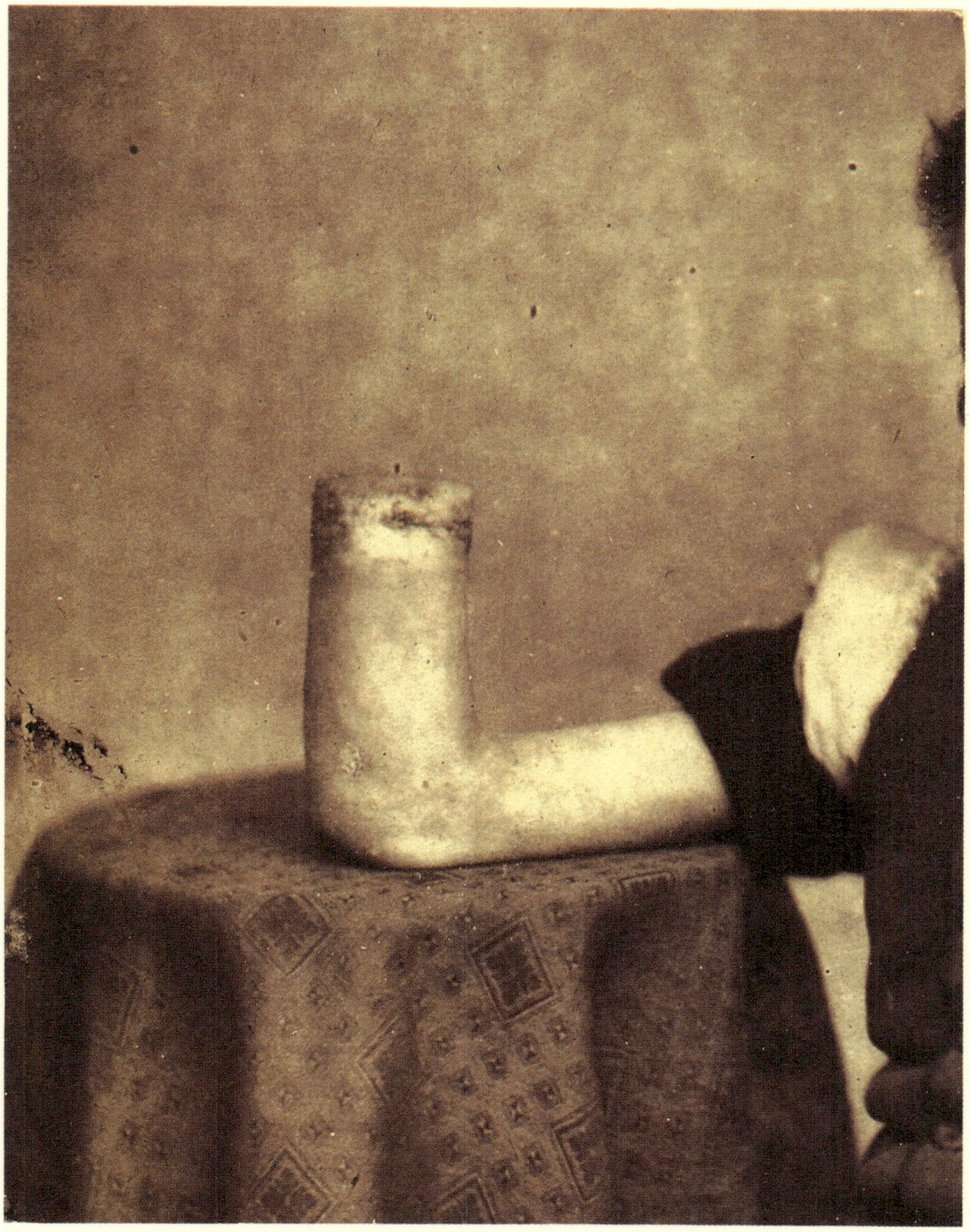

30

Man in Orthopedic Device
Anonymous, United States
9½ x 7¼″, Silver Print
c. 1890

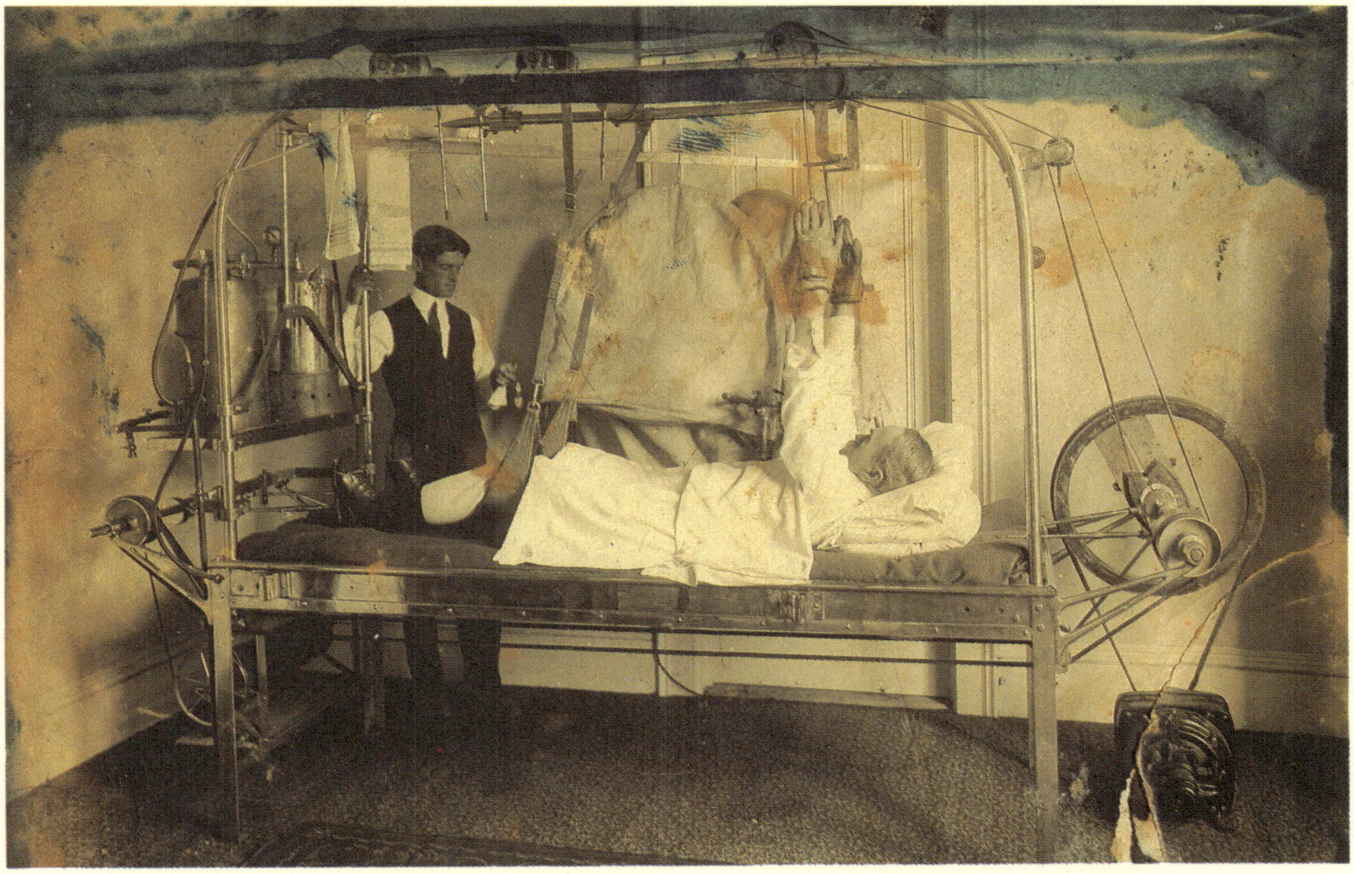

31

Man With Fatty Tumor of the Upper Back
Anonymous, Philadelphia
4 x 5″, Albumen Print
1872

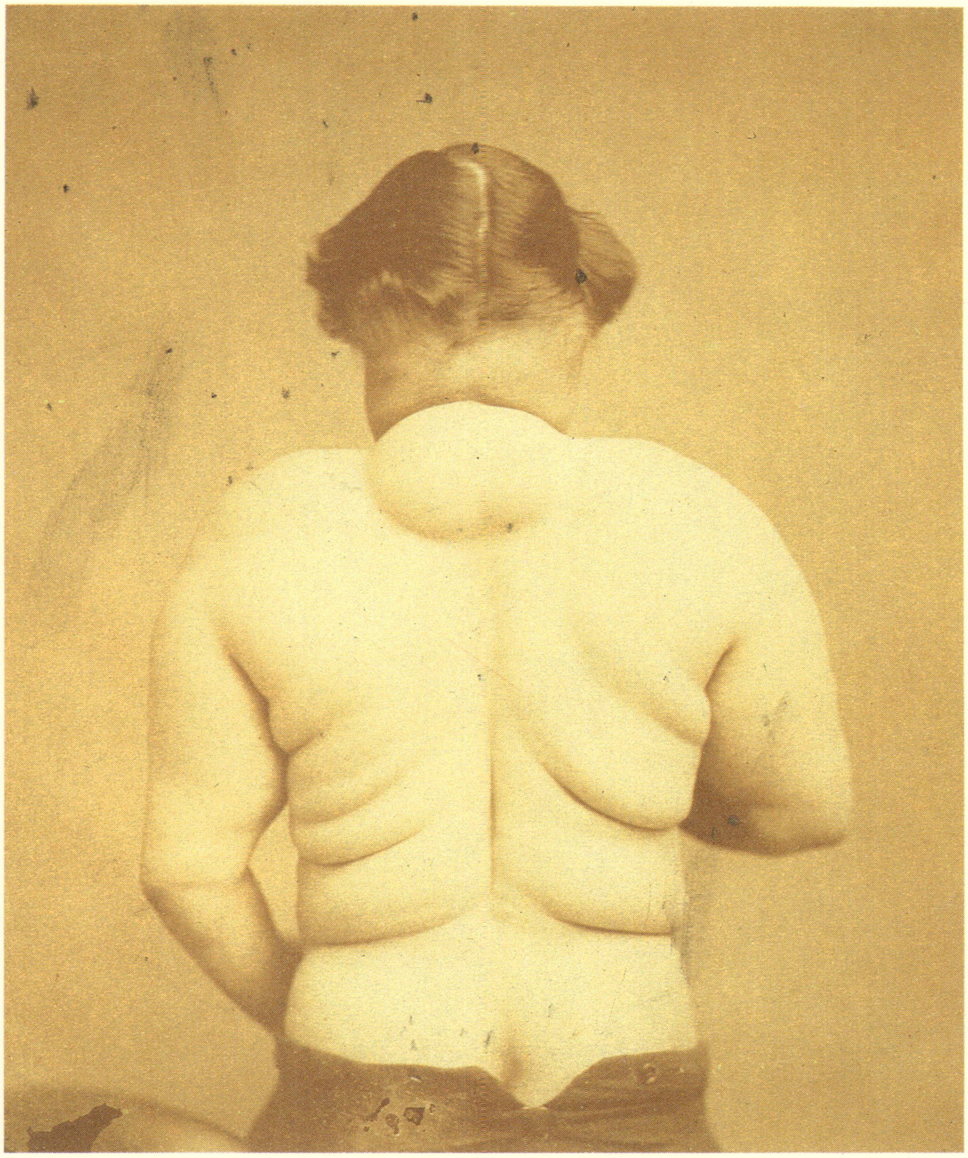

32

THE OPERATION
Anonymous, Baltimore
3¾ x 2¾″, Silver Print
1904

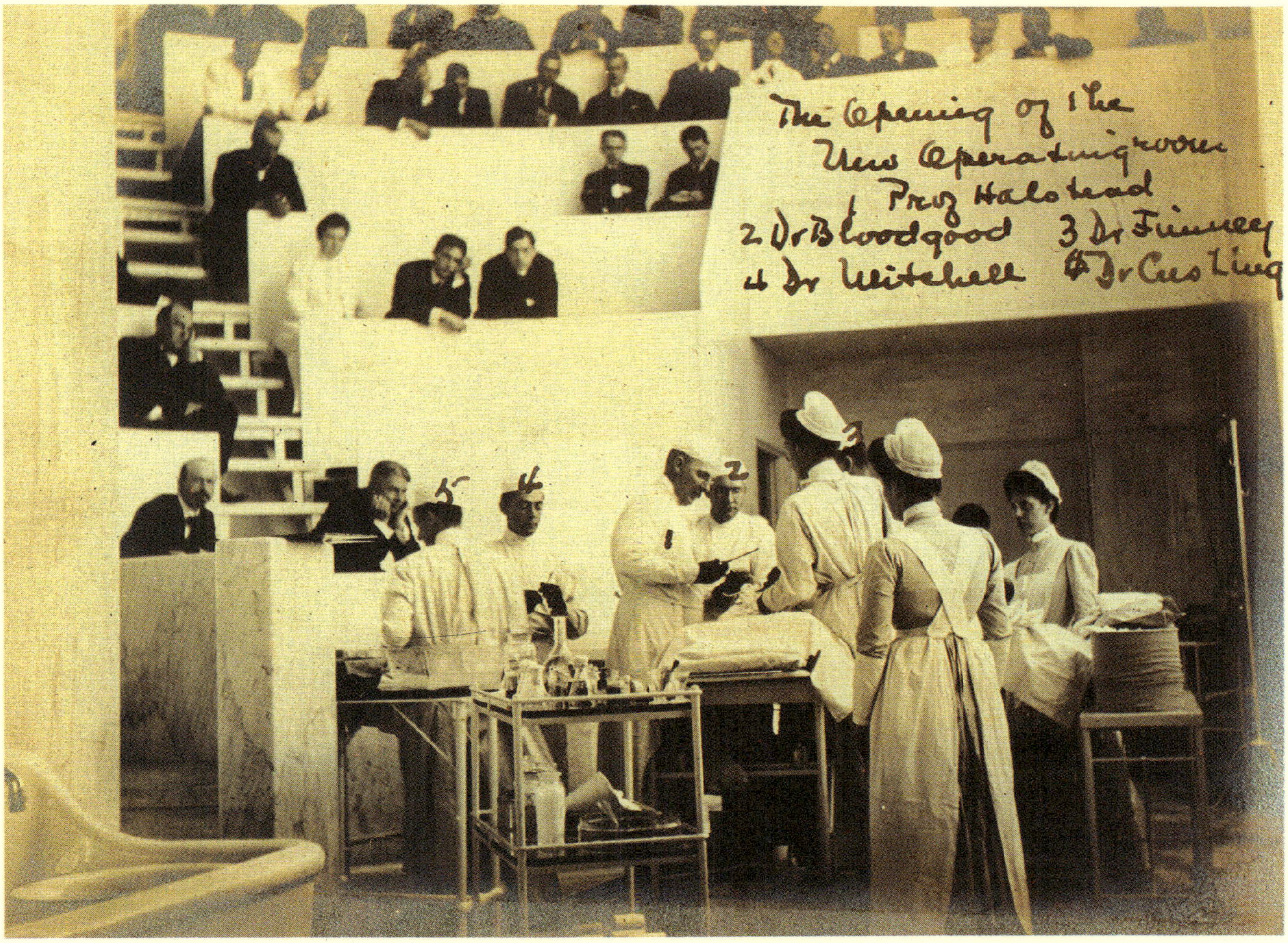
The Opening of the
New Operatingroom
Prof Halstead
2 Dr Bloodgood 3 Dr Finney
4 Dr Mitchell 5 Dr Cushing

33

Irishman In Top Hat With Tumor of the Neck
James Robinson, D.D.S., Dublin, Ireland
4½ x 6½″, Albumen Print
1874

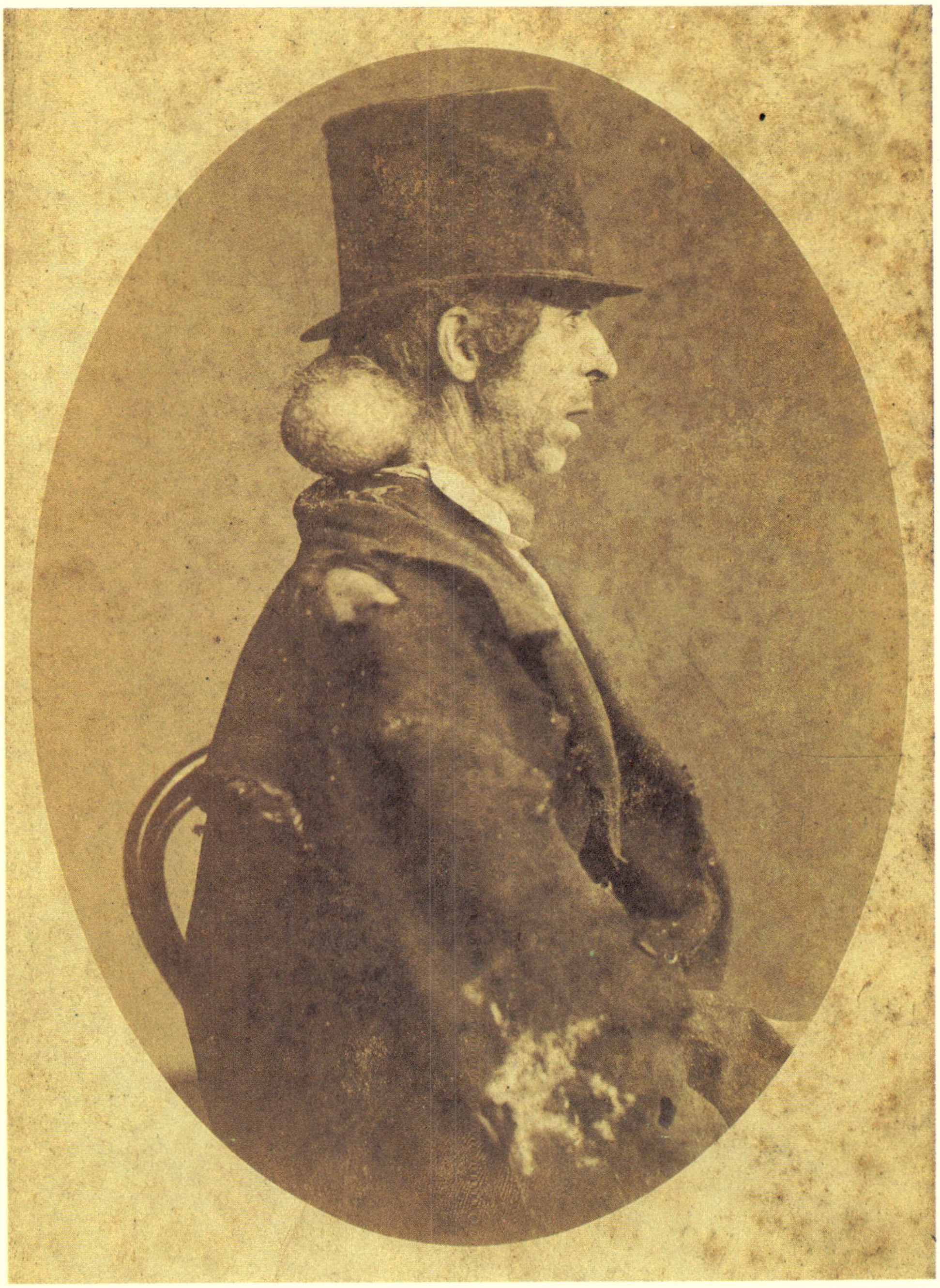

34

Medical Duelling Society
Anonymous, Wurzburg, Germany
5 x 3½″, Photo Postcard
1908

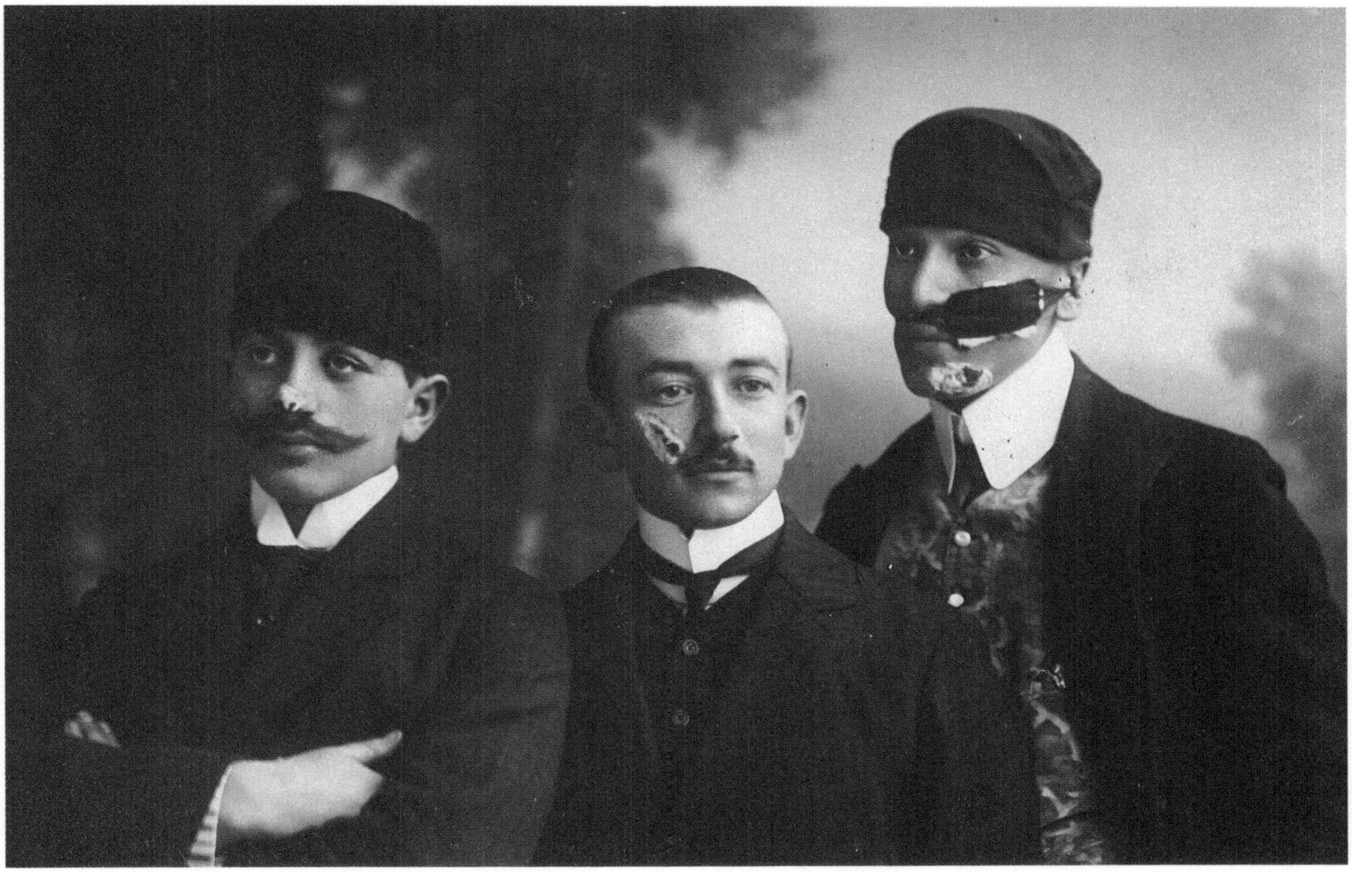

35

Frostbite of the Fingers
O.G. Mason, New York City
2¾ x 4″, Artotype
1885

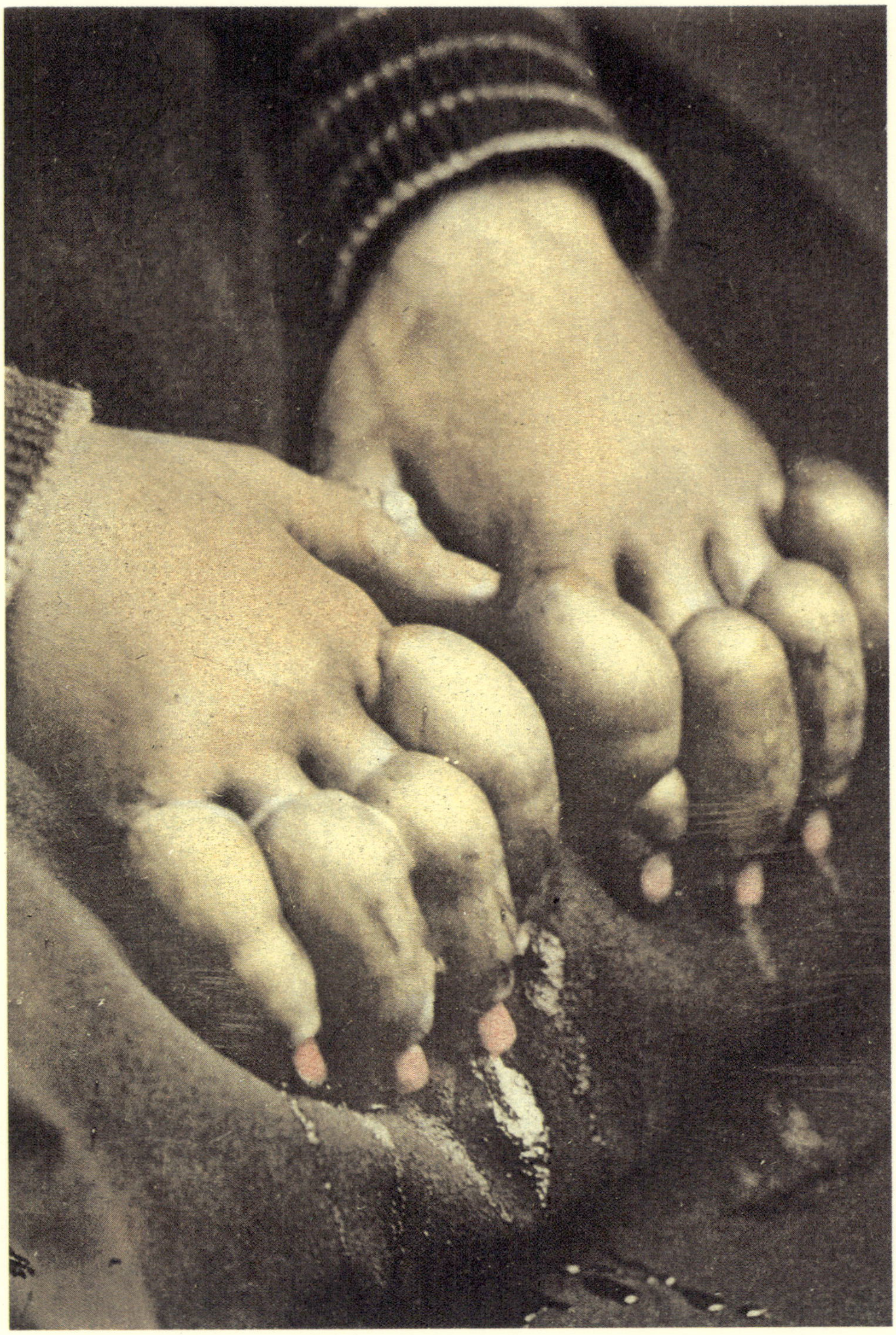

36

Woman With Cured Rodent Cancer
Anonymous, Great Britain
2 x 2½″, Albumen Print
1865

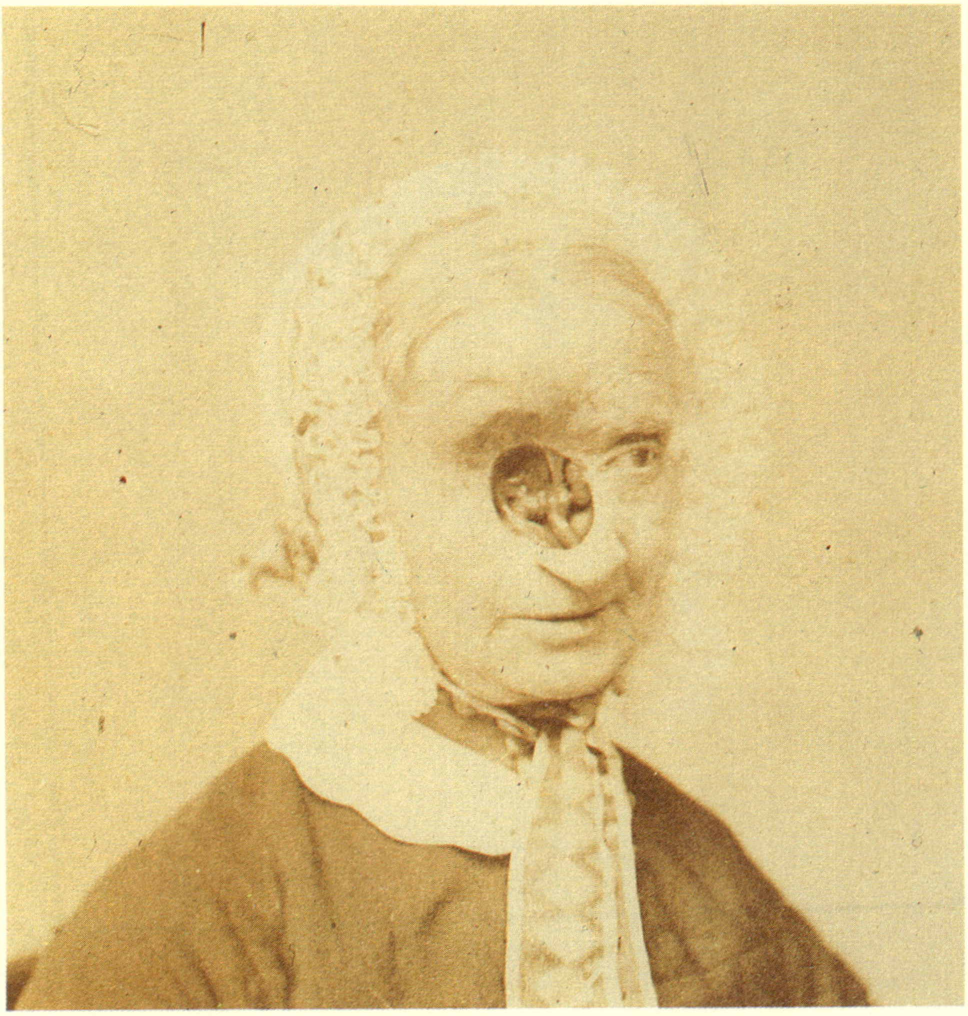

37

Woman Holding Baby With Hare Lip
Thomas North, Dublin, Ireland
4½ x 6½", Albumen Print
1874

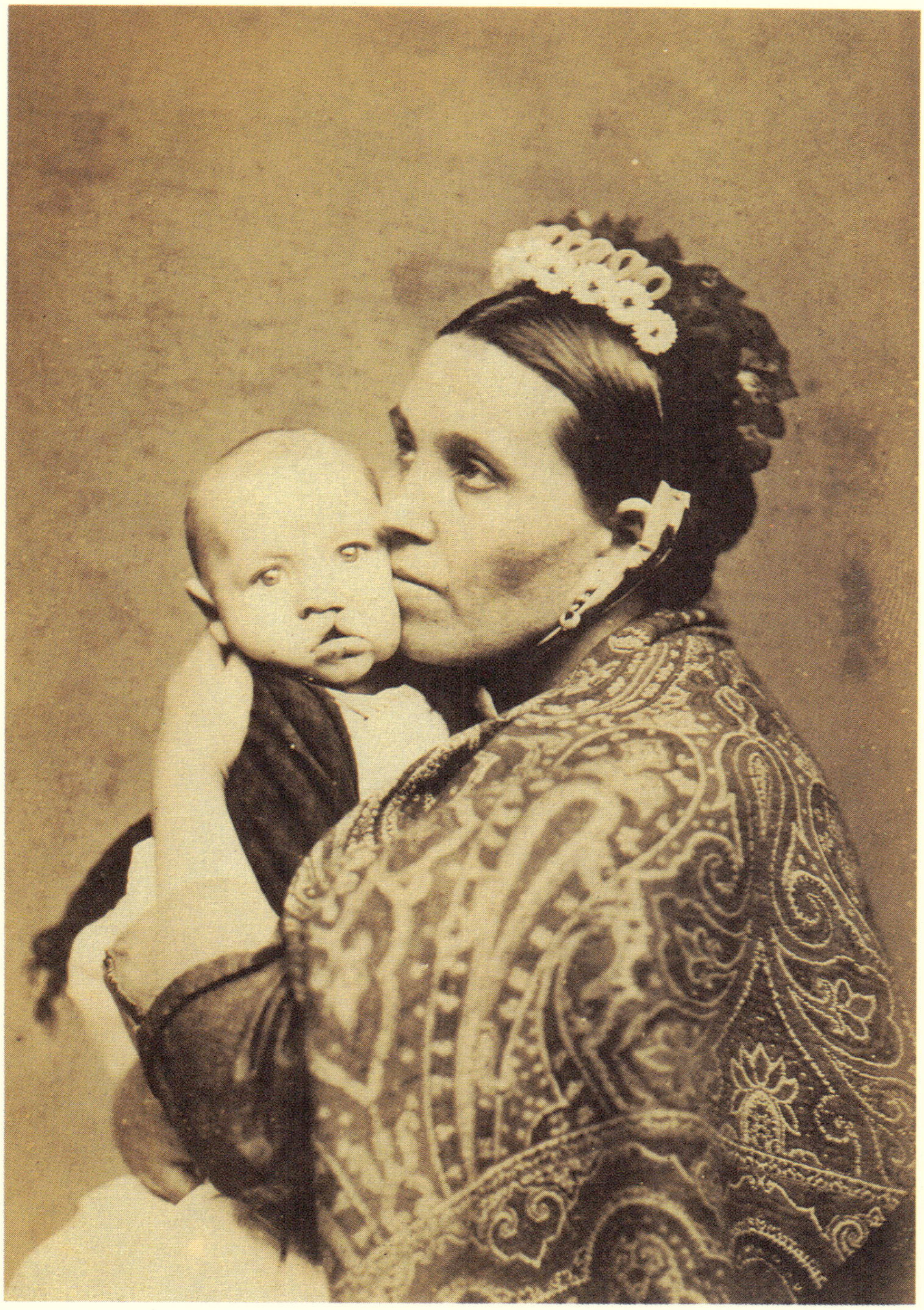

38

NELATON'S PATIENT WITH DERMATOLYSIS
Pierre Petit, Paris, France
3½ x 4½", Albumen Print
1864

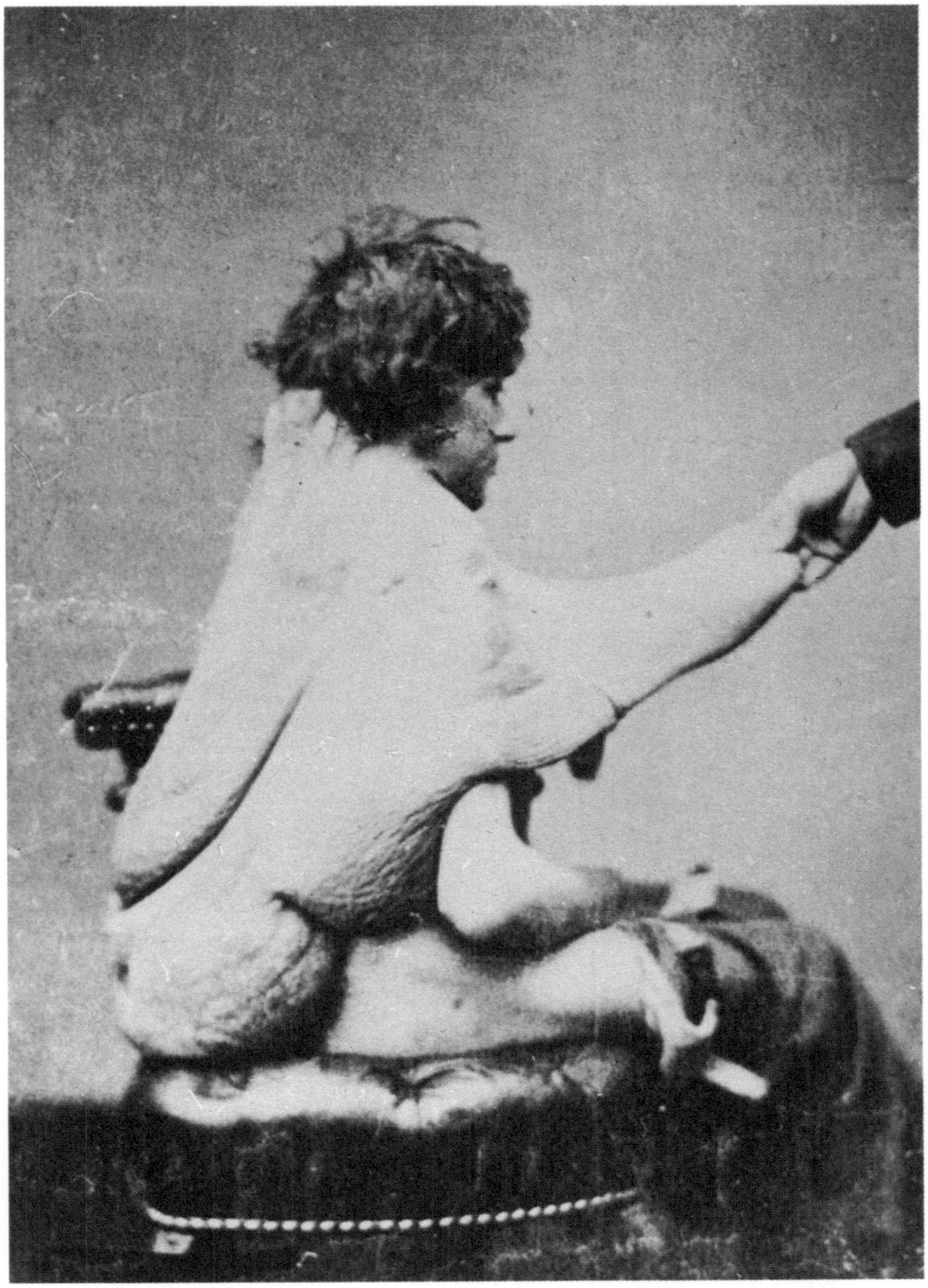

39

Iron Bar Through Skull
Anonymous, Boston
4 x 6½″, Albumen Print
1870

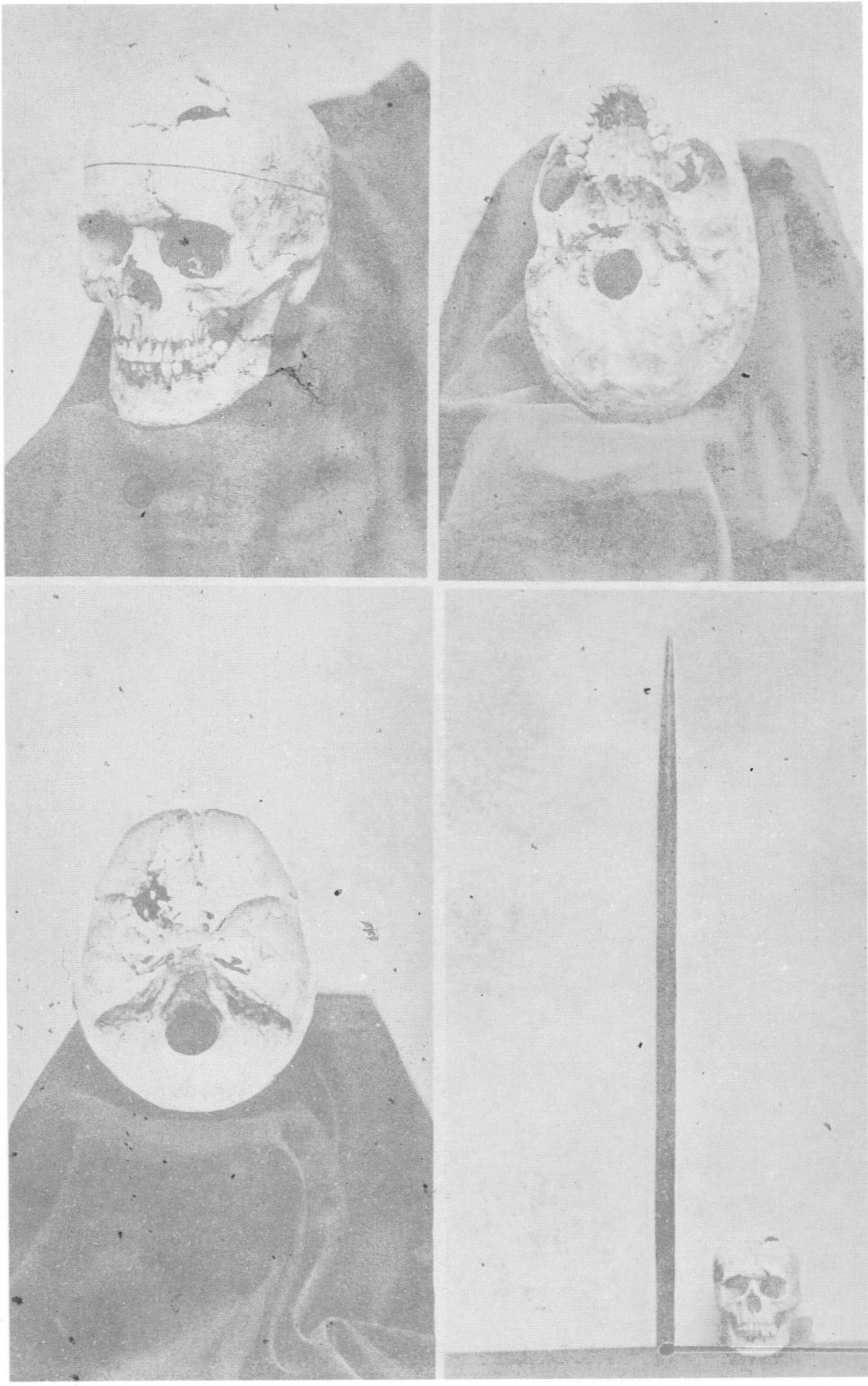

40

Man With Arm Excision and Mirror
James Robinson, D.D.S., Dublin, Ireland
4½ x 6½", Albumen Print
1877

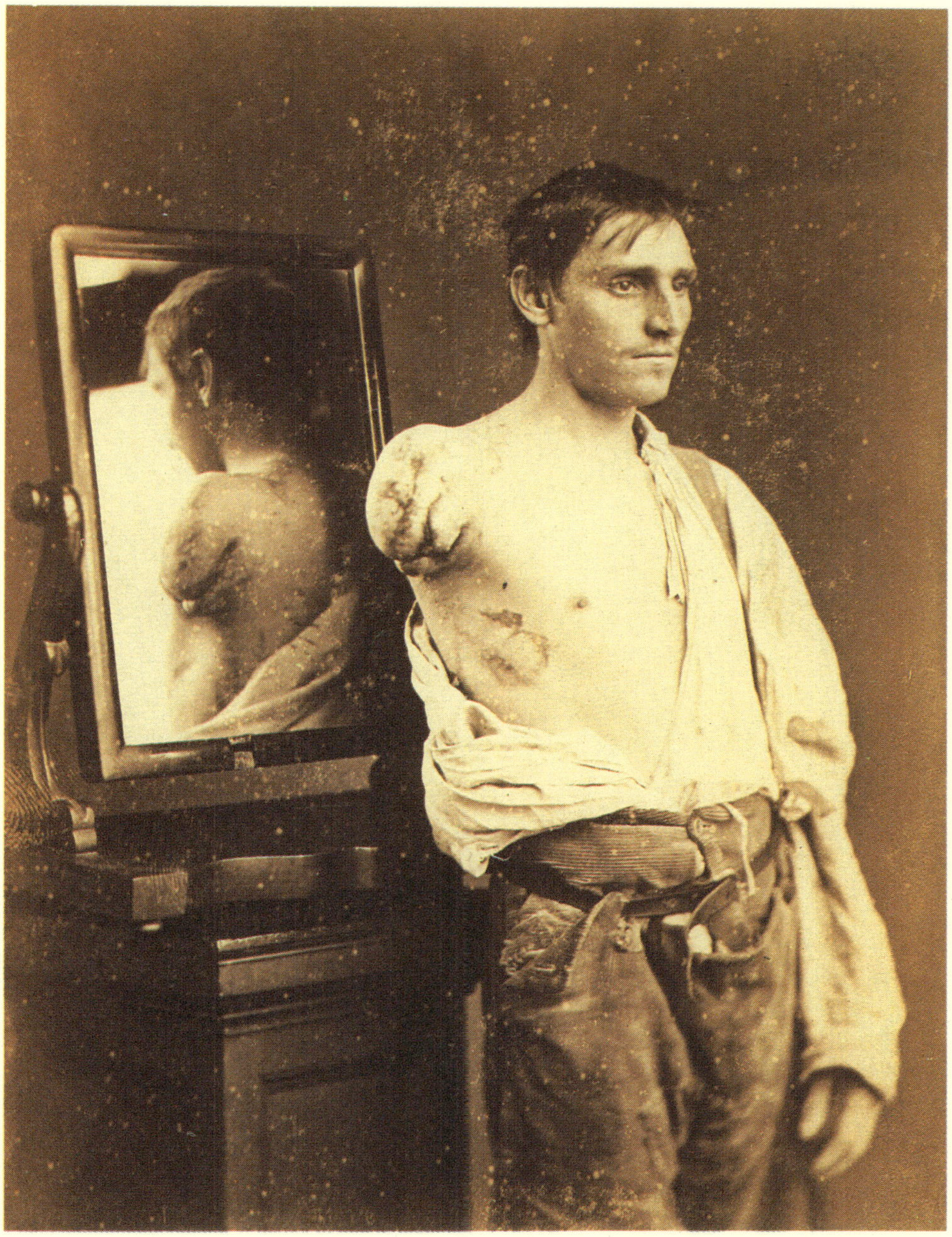

I HAVE ALWAYS BEEN A COLLECTOR, interested in objects for their historical or artistic associations. I am also a physician, and the melding of vocation with avocation led to my collecting medical artifacts.

During the 1970's the collecting of photographs came of age and a more general appreciation of their importance as artistic and historic documents was born. In 1976 I recognized the unique opportunity to collect and preserve medical photographs with the aim of creating an archive that would document the emergence of modern medicine and its effects on our lives. By the end of 1980 the Burns Archive contained over eight thousand vintage photographs taken between the years of 1840 and 1920. It is still growing at the rate of one thousand prints a year. During the span of the collection (1839-1920) the era of modern medicine was born. The discoveries of anaesthesia, antiseptic surgery, the germ theory of disease and x-ray propelled medicine from its dark ages.

I first collected images based on their importance as historical documents but very quickly the artistic strength of this largely unappreciated body of work became evident. I welcome the opportunity to work with Joel-Peter Witkin and Jack Woody in compiling this volume and hope that their aesthetic clarifications and selections will offer a new perspective on the archive to an audience interested in the fine arts.

Stanley B. Burns, M.D. 1987

1

PHYSICIAN WITH HIS MEDICAL BAG
L. Chilton, New York City
2½ x 3¼", Daguerreotype
c. 1847

Posing with the tools of ones trade became a photographic convention during the mid-1840's. Physicians were commonly photographed with a set of medical instruments or with a skull. This daguerreotype shows a physician removing a vial from his medical bag.

The doctor's bag became a symbol of the profession in the twentieth century, but at the time this photograph was taken it was likely to be filled with medications which caused more harm than good. Poisons such as mercury, arsenic and strychnine compounds were standard fare of the day. The violent physical reactions they caused were a part of the so-called "heroic therapy" of the time.

2

DISSECTION SCENE
Byron Reed, Kokimo, Indiana
8½ x 6½", Tintype of Daguerreotype
c. 1844

During the nineteenth and early twentieth centuries having a photographic portrait taken with one's dissection cadaver became an initiation rite of medical practice. This type of "occupational photograph" is the most commonly seen of physicians/students at work. The knowledge of anatomy separated physicians from lay persons, and the photographs provided evidence of a student's entrance into the profession.

3

DR. LETTERMAN EXAMINING A PATIENT
Anonymous, Philadelphia
4¼ x 3¼", Daguerreotype
1849

This image holds a unique place in photographic history as the earliest of a physician examining a patient at bedside. The physician is identified as Jonathan Letterman (1824-1872) and the photograph is dated 1849 when Letterman was in Philadelphia at Jefferson Medical School. He was perhaps directly responsible for saving more lives than any other mid-century American medical practitioner. As Director of the Army of the Potomac his innovations, including new methods of caring for battle-wounded soldiers and more efficient ambulance systems, became the standard around the world.

4

SOUTH AMERICAN INDIAN
WITH A TUMOR OF THE JAW
Anonymous, Caracas, Venezuela
3¼ x 4¼", Daguerreotype
1848

This image is of a South American Indian with a parotid tumor of the jaw. It is the earliest medical photograph from South America and is part of its best documented case history.

Dr. Eliseo Acosta (1819-1879) was the leading pupil and disciple of Dr. Jose Maria Vargas, a friend of Simon Bolivar, who became President of Venezuela in 1835. Vargas and then Acosta were the country's leading surgeons and educators. In this case Acosta was called upon to perform the operation, the first successful removal of a parotid tumor in South America.

5

MOTHER WITH HER DEAD TWINS
Anonymous, United States
2¾ x 3¼", Ambrotype
c. 1855

Since nineteenth century Americans lived with death and disease at home it follows that postmortem photography also came into the home. This unusual example depicts a mother and her recently-born dead twins. Because the infant mortality rate was so high, ranging from thirty to fifty percent, many postmortem photographs from this period are of children. They are of value, historically, as they depict the ravages of diseases long since conquered.

6

DR. SAYRE AND HIS
SUSPENSION DEVICE FOR SCOLIOSIS
Anonymous, London
3½ x 4½", Albumen Print
1877

Tuberculosis, nutritional deficiencies and other diseases made spinal curvature commonplace in the nineteenth century. Dr. Louis A. Sayre of New York's Bellvue Hospital developed a treatment which offered dramatic results. The portable tripod device was given to the patients who suspended themselves from it daily. Every three weeks, as the spine staightened, a new plaster of Paris cast was applied.

This photograph was one of twenty-one appearing in Dr. Sayre's book Spinal Disease and Spinal Curvature and its Treatment.

7

BERNHEIM'S HYPNOTIC TECHNIQUE
Anonymous, Chicago
3¼ x 3¼", Gelatin Print
c. 1895

This image, taken at the Chicago School of Psychiatry, shows a doctor using the method of French physician Hippolyte Marie Bernheim (1840-1919) to conduct a hypnotic treatment.

The pioneer neurologist Jean M. Charcot had used dramatically conducted hypnotic demonstrations in Paris to bring scientific attention to this fledgling therapy. Charcot worked with hysterics, believing that the hypnotic state was capable only in hysterics and that hysteria was an organic brain disease. Bernheim explained both hypnosis and hysteria in purely psychological terms and went a momentous step further by demonstrating that almost anyone could be hypnotized. With posthypnotic suggestion he proved experimentally that unconscious mental information could influence behavior. A young Austrian neurologist, Sigmund Freud, became profoundly interested in Bernheim's concepts, visited his clinic and changed the direction of his own research.

8

BLIND JAPANESE SHIATZU MASSAGE HEALER
Anonymous, Japan
2¼ x 4", Carte de Visite, Tinted Albumen Print
c. 1860

Eastern medical practice has long intrigued western physicians. To this day many successful techniques, acupuncture and acupressure for example, remain unexplained by Occidental science.

Shiatzu massage offered dramatic therapeutic results. Its practitioners were often blind for the Japanese believed the sightless to possess a more sensitive sense of touch which enabled them to detect a variety of ailments through muscle tenseness.

9

Psychiatric Patient in Rag Clothing
Anonymous, France
3½ x 5″, Silver Print
c. 1890

This image is most likely the work of Jean M. Charcot whose *Iconograph Photographique de las Salpetriere* contained hundreds of images of psychiatric patients. Psychiatrists were among the first physicians to systematically photograph patients. These photographs could be used as institutional records, as an aid in capturing those who escaped, and most importantly, in treating patients. Confronted with these frequently shocking images of themselves, patients often responded by trying to avoid looking like they had in their picture.

10

Muybridge Study of Human Motion
Eadweard Muybridge, United States
8½ x 14¼″, Heliotype
1887

During the 1860's doctors, trying to improve the design of artificial limbs needed by tens of thousands of Civil War amputees, studied the physiology of motion. The slow wet-plate process of photography, limited by required long exposures, could not accurately record the mechanics of motion.

In 1877 Eadweard Muybridge, in a demonstration for California gamblers, used twelve cameras triggered by trip-wires to prove that at full stride a horse's four feet are off the ground. He later invented the zoopraxiscope, a device that imparted an illusion of motion to a series of still photographs. It remained the predominant motion viewer until Thomas Edison invented the motion picture camera.

In collaboration with Dr. Francis Xavier Dercum (1856-1931) at the University of Pennsylvania he studied both the normal and abnormal movements of man. The patients of Dercum's neurological institute were brought before his camera to record pathological locomotion and, for the first time, convulsions. In this multiple exposure we see a patient with a gait disorder diagnosed as "spastic diplegia and choreoform and athetoid movement."

Muybridge earned a lasting place in photographic and medical history with his monumental work on animal and human locomotion, taking over 100,000 photographs. In 1887 he published over 20,000 of the photographs in eleven volumes, a work so complete and accurate that no one has attempted to repeat it. His photographs are still used today by artists, photographers and physicians in the study of the body in motion.

11

Dr. Azoux and His Medical Mannequin
Bisson Freres, France
2¼ x 4″, Carte de Visite, Albumen Print
c. 1859

Human dissection was prohibited in many countries until the late nineteenth century. Medical schools used alternative educational aids such as "medical mannequins" to provide their students with meaningful training in anatomy. In 1822 Dr. L. T. Jerome Azoux (1797-1880), the most famous model-maker of the period, developed a special wax which was easy to mold and retained its color. Here he is seen posing with his renowned full-scale model known as "Azoux Man."

12

Old Woman With Eye Tumor
Anonymous, United States
4¼ x 5½″, Albumen Print
c. 1878

Fear of surgery kept many patients from timely care in pre-antiseptic surgery days. Mankind had learned to live with disease and deformity. Eye tumors, however, usually forced those afflicted to seek treatment quickly due to loss of sight and disfigurement. This old woman appears to have been an exception. She suffered most likely from malignant melanoma of the uvea, the most common primary cancerous tumor of the inner eye.

13

Dissected Head In Soup Plate
Howard Brundage, M.D., Columbus, Ohio
7 x 5″, Silver Print
1905

For centuries physicians painstakingly dissected, painted and injected anatomical specimens to demonstrate normal and pathological anatomy. Some dissections took years. Prominent physicians collected such specimens in "medical museums" and passed them from generation to generation.

This turn of the century photograph depicts one such specimen from the anatomy lab of a Columbus medical institution. A head, its posterior portion dissected to show bone, brain and blood vessel relationships, sits in a soup bowl.

14
YOUNG WOMAN WITH
ELEPHANTIASIS FROM SCARLET FEVER
O.G. Mason, New York City
4 x 6¼", Artotype
1878

Most cases of elephantiasis occur in the tropics and are due to parasitic worms that enter the body and block the flow of lymphatic fluids. The girl pictured here suffered not from parasites but from a rare complication of scarlet fever which she contracted at the age of eight. Over the next eleven years, after several bouts of infection and general edema, her legs grew to the grotesque proportions seen here. Her body remained normal above the waist.

15
ERYSIPELAS INFECTION AFTER THUMB AMPUTATION
Reed B. Bontecou, M.D., Washington D.C.
3½ x 3½", Albumen Print
1865

Reed Brockway Bontecou, M.D. was surgeon in charge of Harewood U.S. Army General Hospital. With three thousand beds it was the largest Federal General Hospital of the Civil War. In 1862 Dr. William Hammond, then Surgeon General, ordered the collecting of medical specimens and photographs of interesting cases which were to be sent to his innovative Army Medical Museum and used in teaching the Army's thousands of new physicians about treatment of war wounds.

An avid photographer, Dr. Bontecou contributed one album of almost six hundred carte de visite sized photographs and several other albums, each containing approximately one hundred 4½ x 6½" images. His work became a foundation of the Army Medical Museum which developed into the Armed Forces Institute of Pathology. It presently houses the world's largest collection of reference pathological photography.

All wounds became infected during the Civil War years and most visible signs of infection were considered little more than part of the healing process. There were, however, five "abnormal infections" feared because of the devastation they caused. These included tetanus, chronic bone infection (osteomyelitis), pyemia (septicemia), hospital gangrene and erysipelis, the latter three becoming known as "hospitalism."

Private Shadle was wounded at the Battle of Petersburg, one of the final battles of the war. His wounded thumb was amputated at a field station. He was then sent to Harewood Hospital where he contracted erysipelas. The infection spread through his arm and shoulder causing the disfigurement seen here and threatening his life. Treated with frequent incisions and liberal dousing with tincture of ferric chloride, Shadle survived and was discharged on June 1, 1865.

16
HOSPITAL GANGRENE
Reed B. Bontecou, Washington D.C.
4½ x 6½", Albumen Print
1865

This was the first published photograph of a patient with hospital gangrene, one of the dread triad of diseases known as "hospitalism." Because this infection was so sensitive to the principles of washing, cleanliness and antiseptics it disappeared in the early antiseptic era and its bacteriological cause has never been discovered. It is now hard to understand how it could have spread like wildfire through hospital wards.

A few physicians did recognize its nature. Civil War surgeons Drs. W.W. Keen and M. Goldsmith isolated their cases, washed linens and used iodine and bromine as disinfectants. They had a surprising understanding of contagious cross contamination and its prevention. Unfortunately their work was not generally accepted by their peers and it remained for England's Joseph Lister to establish the principles of antiseptic surgery in 1867.

Twenty-year-old James Stokes, Private, Co. H, 185th New York, was wounded at Gravelly Run, Virginia on March 29, 1865 with a bullet to the right forearm and elbow. On April 3rd doctors made a one inch incision over the elbow to look for the bullet. Almost a month later the nearly healed wound became gangrenous. The wound was then treated with further incisions and drenched with turpentine and kerosine. Stokes survived and was discharged on July 5,1865, his elbow enlarged and frozen (ankylosed) in the position photographed.

17

Sutured Gunshot Wound of the Upper Arm

Reed B. Bontecou, M.D., Washington D.C.
4½ x 6½", Albumen Print
1865

A superficial bullet wound runs across this soldier's chest with one hole appearing directly in the center of his chest. The bullet passed across his chest and shattered the humerus of his left arm. Of 8,245 such fractures of the humerus treated surgically, more than half were amputated. Thousands of others were treated by resection or excision of the bone.

Nineteen-year-old Corporal E.M. Bostwick, Co. H, 52nd New York Calvary, was wounded on April 1, 1865. He underwent immediate surgery by his regimental surgeon, S.F. Kingston, and had three inches of humerus excised. Bostwick was one of only 326 patients to survive such an operation.

18

Amputation at the Hip Joint

Reed B. Bontecou, M.D., Washington D.C.
4½ x 6½", Albumen Print
1865

The most serious operation attempted during the Civil War era was the amputation of a leg at the hip. It involved the disarticulation of the largest bone in the body from the largest joint. Blood loss, shock and infection claimed most patients' lives. Of the sixty-six war-wounded patients to undergo this operation only eleven survived, a mortality rate of eighty-three percent.

Although this image is unidentified, a study of the eleven surviving men and their photographs indicates this patient is Private Lewis Francis, Co. I, 14th New York. He received fifteen bayonet stabs on July 1, 1861 at Bull Run, one of the first battles of the war. The most serious of these opened his right knee joint. He was taken prisoner and placed in a Confederate hospital where a mid-thigh amputation was performed. In 1862 he was "exchanged" and went home to New York. Because of infection what remained of his leg was amputated at the hip. Private Francis survived the operation but, like many war-wounded veterans, was plagued with sinuses and ulcers in the wound area. He died on May 31, 1874, the day after he marched, with the aid of crutches, in Brooklyn's (Decoration) Memorial Day Parade.

19

Gunshot Wound of the Hand

Reed B. Bontecou, M.D., Washington D.C.
4½ x 6½", Albumen Print
1865

Robert Freyer, Co. G, 52nd New York, was wounded during the battle of Hatchers Run, Virginia on March 25, 1865. Three fingers were amputated in the field and his wound healed cleanly. Most Civil War photographs of wounded are posed casually and with an identification board. Here the photographer formally dressed and posed his subject.

20

Arm Amputation By Flap Technique

Reed B. Bontecou, M.D., Washington D.C.
4½ x 6½", Albumen Print
1865

Of the two styles of amputation common during the Civil War the "flap" technique was preferred by most surgeons. Although more tissue had to be sacrificed to provide the large flaps, it left a better stump than the circular technique. Here John Murphy of Company K, 87th Maryland Volunteers, displays his flap technique amputation. The swollen limb indicates that infection may be present.

21

Bone Excision

Reed B. Bontecou, M.D., Washington D.C.
4½ x 6½", Albumen Print
1864

One of the most functionally mutilating operations performed during the Civil War was bone excision. Rather than amputate a limb that had suffered a bony fracture from gunshot or other trauma, part or all of the bone was removed. The patient was often left with a useless appendage dangling from the body.

Sergeant T. Newell, Co. C, 112th New York Volunteers, suffered a gunshot wound June 1, 1864 at the battle of Cold Harbor, Virginia. A resection of the entire upper third of the left humerus was performed at a field hospital and he healed without complication. Sergeant Newell's sagging arm demonstrates the missing bone. A photographer's head rest holds his useless but still attached limb. In 1874 Newell wrote the pension board. "I have use of my hand, but cannot put it to my mouth. Only as I take the other hand I can place it on the table and hold my fork, but cannot feed myself with it...my arm is but little account yet I would not have it off for anything."

22
GUNSHOT WOUND OF THE HEAD
Reed B. Bontecou, M.D., Washington D.C.
4½ x 6½", Albumen Print
1865

Surviving a bullet wound to the head, neck or face during the Civil War was unusual. One battlefield study indicated that over eighty percent of those killed in the field, but only eleven percent of the wounded, suffered from head, neck or chest wounds. As all wounds became infected in those days even the slightest head or scalp wound could prove fatal, the infection easily penetrating the tissues protecting the brain. In rare cases patients miraculously survived devastating wounds and lived their lives with brains visibly pulsating beneath a scarred meningeal membrane.

Corporal Ansdell Beam, Co. I, 26th Michigan Volunteers was wounded at the battle of Farmersville, Virginia on April 6, 1985. The bullet glanced off of but fractured his skull. On this photograph surgeons have highlighted in red ink the tissue damage and suspected path of the bullet.

Although Corporal Beam "had many symptoms of brain disturbance," his wound healed and he was discharged on July 6, 1865. While many soldiers posed wearing their division or corps badges, Beam is pictured wearing the sign of his international fraternal brotherhood organization, The Masons.

23
EMBALMING SURGEON
Matthew Brady
3¼ x 3¼", Albumen Print
1864

Matthew Brady revolutionized photojournalism by taking his camera onto the battlefield and bringing back images of the war which found their way into the homes and conciousness of America. Brady and his fellow photographers produced thousands of images of the Civil War as stereophotographs, until then a form of nineteenth century home-entertainment. This popular image of Richard Burr, M.D., embalming surgeon of the Army of the Potomac, at work certainly brought home the finality of war.

Nonmilitary embalmers often followed the troops into battle, offering their services at exorbitant prices. As most of the units were formed locally and often consisted of life-long friends, one's comrades assumed the financial burden.

24
A MORNING'S WORK
Reed B. Bontecou, M.D., Washington D.C.
6 x 4", Albumen Print
1865

This photograph graphically documents Civil War devastation. More than 625,000 men died, one of every four that fought. In addition, more than 400,000 were wounded. Infections, chronic diarrhea and dysentery killed tens of thousands in the years following the war as a ravaged generation and a young nation continued to pay the cost of war.

25
ANDERSONVILLE PRISONER
Matthew Brady, Washington D.C.
3¼ x 3¼", Albumen Print
c. 1865

On the back of this stereophotograph (war view #4009) is this testimony: "Benjamin T. Daughtery, a Private in Co. K, 31st Illinois Volunteers swears that he enlisted on August 10, 1861, that he was taken prisoner at Hillsborough, Mississippi on February 19, 1864... was taken to Andersonville, Georgia in April of 1864 and was exchanged March 1, 1865...and that he or his fellow prisoners were not provided with any shelter, but were exposed to the inclemency of the weather; and were obliged to dig holes in the ground to protect them in some slight degree from the cold. And by reason of such exposure and the other cruel and inhuman treatment... his feet have come off above the ankle and he has been reduced to his present condition. Sworn this 28th day of April, 1865."

26
BONE FRAGMENTS
Reed B. Bontecou, M.D., Washington D.C.
2¼ x 4", Carte de Visite, Albumen Prints
1864

Dr. Bontecou's photographic record of Civil War wounds and treatments, successful and failed, was unparalleled in its era and proved a useful tool for the next generation of surgeons. This page of mounted photographs is the last in Bontecou's carte de visite "Harewood Hospital Album of Wounded Soldiers."

27

WOMAN WITH NECK LESIONS

O.G. Mason, New York City

4¾ x 6¼", Artotype

c. 1881

"The recognition of syphilis is the most important features of dermatological diagnosis" wrote George Henry Fox in his 1881 treatise, "Photographic illustrations of Cutaneous Syphilis." Although syphilis can mimic most known diseases, in the skin it is most easily recognized since syphilis can cause every possible type of skin eruption.

This patient's condition came about when dead skin accumulated on syphilitic sores, giving a scaly, pearlized appearance. The friction of the patient's clothing further irritated the lesions.

28

GIRL WITH LARGE FOOT JUMPING ROPE

Dewitt, Scranton, Pennsylvania

4 x 5½", Cabinet Card

c. 1895

Until the twentieth century people often lived with gross deformities of the limbs. Surgery and its accompanying infections could result in worse disfigurement or even death. Development of modern microsurgical, orthopedic and plastic surgical procedures now allow even the most severe cases to be treated and most patients to live near-normal lives.

Posing with a jumping rope serves only to exaggerate this young girl's foot deformity. Perhaps the intended message was that with her new orthopedic boot she had more normal function of her foot.

29

AMPUTATED ARM CURED BY EARTH DRESSING

Anonymous, Philadelphia

3 x 4", Albumen Print

1869

One fascinating aspect of medical discovery is that, occasionally, great ideas and advances lay hidden in old books and journals. Open minds and new technology are sometimes necessary to understand and implement the discoveries of the past.

Dr. Addinell Hewson published *Earth as a Topical Application in Surgery* in 1872. In it he describes his treatment of wounds and operative cases by application of earth to the wound, and the accompanying acceleration of the healing process. He details ninety-three cases including ulcers, burns, gunshot wounds and operations such as mastectomy. All wounds were dressed with his special dirt, and all healed quickly. Hewson attributed this healing to the action of ozone, deoxygenation and released ammonia. More likely any inhibition of infection was due to the presence of naturally occurring antibacterial agents, such as bacitracin, in the soil.

The patient pictured above had suffered from osteomyelitis of the wrist for eight months prior to treatment by Dr. Hewson. After four days of applying earth dressings his wound was free of infection. A new amputation was performed and fifteen days later, when this photograph was taken, there was no apparent infection.

Unfortunately for Hewson, his work appeared before bacteriological concepts of disease were discovered by Pasteur. At the same time Lister's antiseptic surgical technique was being promoted and widely accepted by surgeons. Packing wounds with dirt made no sense to a profession recently convinced of the necessity for cleanliness in their work. Had Hewson's findings been taken more seriously and evaluated by open minds, the age of antibiotics might have dawned a half-century sooner.

30

MAN IN ORTHOPEDIC DEVICE

Anonymous, United States

9½ x 7¼", Silver Print

c. 1890

Like other types of surgery, orthopedics was not always dominated by physicians. As late as the nineteenth century bone setters called "Rabonteurs" provided treatment for fractures. The secrets of these Rabonteurs were kept within their families and passed from generation to generation. Only when Hugh Owen Thomas (1834-1891), a member of the most prominent bone setting family and a Rabonteur, became a physician were these secrets made available to the medical profession.

Orthopedic treatment during the nineteenth century was usually limited to manipulation with mechanical devices, braces and, after the development of plaster of Paris bandage in 1852, casts. This era of orthopedic history is known as the "strap and buckle era." The device pictured here is one of many contraptions used in treating the musculoskeletal system.

31
MAN WITH FATTY TUMOR OF THE UPPER BACK
Anonymous, Philadelphia
4 x 5″, Albumen Print
1872

This patient presented a rare symmetrical expression of subcutaneous fatty tumors of his back. Dr. A.C.W. Beedher published the image and case history in the "Photographic Review of Medicine and Surgery"; a pioneering medical journal that presented photographs of the most dramatic and extreme cases of disease.

32
THE OPERATION
Anonymous, Baltimore
3¾ x 2¾″, Silver Print
1904

Modern American medicine and teaching practices began at John Hopkins Hospital. The residency system of medical training, now used worldwide, began here. New medical and surgical standards were established by Doctors Osler, Kelly, Halstead and Welch. Eventually their accomplishments brought Europeans to America for training.

An important event in the history of John Hopkins was the opening of a new surgical amphitheater on October 5, 1904. John Hopkins' finest surgeons were assembled for the event and a photographer was hired to record the proceedings. The photographs were later mounted in souvenir albums and presented to important hospital personnel. In this photograph William Steward Halstead, M.D., the father of modern American surgery, wears the rubber gloves which he developed.

33
IRISHMAN IN TOP HAT WITH TUMOR OF THE NECK
James Robinson, D.D.S., Dublin, Ireland
4½ x 6½″, Albumen Print
1874

During the nineteenth century a patient's social status often dictated the manner in which he was clinically photographed. In nearly every instance patients appeared full-figure, dressed in their street clothes. Draping of patients was rare and usually confined to the upper classes. The diseased part of the body was exposed and photographed without regard to modern concepts of modesty.

As doctors were better able to diagnose and isolate disease, improved medical photography became possible. By the twentieth century the clinical convention of carefully draping all patients, regardless of social standing, was firmly established. Photographers made every effort to isolate wounds and diseased parts. Recording the disease had become more important than photographing the patient.

This photograph was taken by dental surgeon turned photographer, James Robinson. It appeared as an engraving in the "Dublin Journal of Medical Science," Vol. LX, 1875.

34
MEDICAL DUELLING SOCIETY
Anonymous, Wurzburg, Germany
5 x 3½″, Photo Postcard
1908

Duelling, since its recognized inception in 501 A.D., had engaged royalty, men of honor, intellectuals and even physicians. During the nineteenth and early twentieth centuries in Germany, hundreds of "Korps", or duelling societies, were formed and they became an intrinsic part of German life. The wounds sustained were considered badges of courage to be proudly displayed and a sabre scar across the face became almost a German trademark.

This photograph shows three medical students who had just returned from a duel. The photograph was taken and sent home as a proud demonstration of their initiation into the Germanic order.

35
FROSTBITE OF THE FINGERS
O.G. Mason, New York City
2¾ x 4″, Artotype
1885

Cutaneous insult is familiar to many of us from cooking burns or sunburn. Less common is cutaneous inflammation caused by cold. As with burns, blistered skin forms tense bullae and ulceration may occur. When circulation is restored fingers can eventually regain a normal appearance though some discoloration and scarring may remain.

Dr. George H. Fox published this image in *Photographic Illustrations of Skin Disease.*

36

WOMAN WITH CURED RODENT CANCER

Anonymous, Great Britain

2 x 2½", Albumen Print

1865

In 1867 a London surgeon, Clarles Moore, published his text "Rodent Cancer" noting "A disease more repulsive and distressing can hardly be conceived...Commencing in some trifling manner in the skin it spreads in all directions...slowly it grows and ulcerates...but never heals."

Dr. Moore cured this woman with several months use of a solution of arsenic, iodine and mercury, followed by chloride of zinc paste. We now know rodent cancer as Basal Cell Carcinoma, a common skin cancer often related to exposure to the sun.

37

WOMAN HOLDING BABY WITH HARE LIP

Thomas North, Dublin, Ireland

4½ x 6½", Albumen Print

1874

Thomas North worked on photographer's row in Dublin and became associated with James Robinson & Son and their work with medical photography. North took this pre-operative photograph in 1874 while serving as medical photographer for Dublin hospitals and the Royal College of Surgeons. It is one of an extensive collection of "cabinet card" photographs taken by North and James Robinson now in the Burns Archive.

38

NELATON'S PATIENT WITH DERMATOLYSIS

Pierre Petit, Paris, France

3½ x 4½", Albumen Print

1864

One of the most unusual disfiguring diseases of mankind is dermatolysis, now known as cutis laxa. The disease destroys skin elasticity causing it to grow and fall in lax, massive folds. It can effect any part of the body and is caused by a defect in copper metabolism and/or an inherited recessive gene.

This case may be the most extreme ever encountered. The patient, a twenty-eight year old Parisian man, sought the assistance of France's most able surgeon, Auguste Nelaton (1807-1873). The huge folds of skin were isolated using nineteen needles with strong cord as suture and the entire cloak-like mass was removed. It weighed twenty-five pounds. The patient acquired a postoperative infection and died six days after surgery.

39

IRON BAR THROUGH SKULL

Anonymous, Boston

4 x 6½", Albumen Print

1870

This photograph of a skull and thirteen pound iron bar is a legacy from one of the most bizarre medical case histories ever recorded. On September 13, 1848, twenty-five-year-old Phineas Gage was placing explosives with a tamping rod when the charge exploded prematurely. The rod was sent through Gage's skull, exited the top of his head and landed several yards away.

Gage did not die as expected. The next day Dr. John Harow examined his wound and protruding brain. Concerned about foreign matter, Harow "passed one index finger down its whole length from above, the other freely upward from below, 'til they touched."

Despite primitive treatments, hemorrhaging, and even development of a brain abscess Gage survived and, two and one-half months after he was wounded, went home suffering only minimal neurological damage. In spite of the loss of his left eye, he returned to his rugged frontier life, traveling to South America where he became a stagecoach driver.

On May 20, 1861, almost thirteen years after his injury, Gage died after suffering convulsions. His skull and the iron bar were sent to Boston's Warren Anatomical Museum where they remain on display. Despite authenticated documentation and physical evidence the incident defies belief.

40

MAN WITH ARM EXCISION AND MIRROR

James Robinson, D.D.S., Dublin, Ireland

4½ x 6½", Albumen Print

1877

Using a mirror to reflect another view of a wound was a mid-nineteenth century photographic convention. Most frequently used in postoperative amputation cases, it allowed a better perspective of treatment results. This image appeared as an engraving with a case history in the "Dublin Journal of Medical Science," Vol. LXV, 1878.

I would like to thank those individuals who over the past decade have helped me promote early medical photography as art and cultural history. Their energy, resources and media affiliations have been instrumental in helping the Burns Archive grow and reach an ever increasing audience. In addition, I want to express my deepest appreciation to the following men and women whose ideas and support have so often before gone unheralded: The late Alfred Angrist, M.D., Stephen Brennan, Sara Cleary, Barbara Kirshenblatt-Gimblett, Kinten E. Hall, Marvin Heifferman, Yvonne Korshak, Ph.D., Max Koslow, Diane Laks, Nancy R. Larsen, Emily Madoff, Robert Miller, Sharon Romm, M.D., Carrie Stieber, Alfred Vogl.

Stanley B. Burns, M.D., 1987

Joel-Peter Witkin's photographs have recently been included in the George Eastman House traveling exhibition "Images of Excellence" and the Whitney Museum's "Twentieth Century American Master Photographs." The photographs are in the permanent collections of the Museum of Modern Art, New York, Victoria and Albert Museum, London, and the Centre George Pompidou, Paris. In 1985 a monograph, *Joel-Peter Witkin,* was published by Twelvetrees Press. He resides in Albuquerque, New Mexico.

Stanley B. Burns, M.D. is founder of the Burns Archive and author of *Early Medical Photography in America 1839-1883*, published in 1984. He is also author of *The Gallery of Medical History,* a quarterly journal published by Bristol Laboratories. In 1984 the exhibition "In the picture of Health; Selections from the Burns Archive" was curated by Marvin Heifferman and shown at The Center for Experimental Photographic Art in Buffalo, New York. Dr. Burns is an ophthalmologist practicing in New York City.

The first edition of
MASTERPIECES OF MEDICAL PHOTOGRAPHY
is limited to 3000 casebound copies

Plates are printed four color on uncoated paper
Typeface is Baskerville Medium
Design is by Jack Woody
Printed and bound in Hong Kong
for
TWELVETREES PRESS
POST OFFICE BOX 188
PASADENA, CALIFORNIA 91102

ISBN 0-942642-21-X